The Case Against Hysterectomy

What every woman – and man – should know about the
operations to remove the womb and cervix (hysterectomy),
and the ovaries (oophorectomy)

SANDRA SIMKIN

An Imprint of HarperCollins*Publishers*

This book is dedicated to all those women in their twenties and thirties, and those who are still in their teens, who have not yet attracted the attention of gynaecologists. By reading it I hope that they will demand better treatment and not be the victims of unnecessary operations in the way that their mothers and grandmothers have been.

Pandora
An Imprint of HarperCollinsPublishers
77-85 Fulham Palace Road,
Hammersmith, London W6 8JB

Published by Pandora 1996
10 9 8 7 6 5 4 3 2 1

© Sandra Simkin

Sandra Simkin asserts the moral right to
be identified as the author of this work

A catalogue record for this book
is available from the British Library

ISBN 0 04 440978 8

Printed and bound in Great Britain by
Caledonian International Book Manufacturing Ltd, Glasgow

Contents

Acknowledgements

The author acknowledges the help of journalist Caroline Richmond who provided much of the medical research material; Patricia Nolan, a nurse currently working in the NHS and a retired surgeon who have provided further anecdotal and research material; a gynaecologist currently working in the NHS and a medical sociologist, who reviewed the manuscript. The views expressed in this book are my own.

Introduction

Hysterectomy is consistently portrayed by gynaecologists as being of value to women. Through the profession's effective public relations machinery their brochures paint a rosy picture of the operation and its outcome. It is presented as being the cure for everything from backache to stress incontinence or other bladder problems; in addition it will rid women of heavy menstrual bleeding – which naturally no woman wants – and, with no evidence to back it up, gynaecologists will tell you that, what's more, women are very happy with their hysterectomies.

What they deliberately do not spell out, however, is that along with your womb you will also lose some sense of your identity as a woman. And this sense of loss will stay with you long after the scars have disappeared – possibly for the rest of your life. You will also experience a sense of emptiness and, for many women, a loss of libido and sexual functioning. In fact, hysterectomy means the end of sex for many women although it is never presented this way. If hysterectomy is what a woman wants, then no one should stand in her way. But no other person, especially a male gynaecologist, has the right to make that decision for her, nor to persuade her to have the operation without being in full possession of the facts.

In researching this book, I have spoken to many women and studied medical papers on the operation's psychological and emotional consequences. Medical studies reveal a high ratio of women requiring post-operative counselling with a small percentage needing long-stay hospital treatment.

There is a growing and alarming trend for performing this operation on women in their twenties and thirties; for removing perfectly healthy ovaries from women under the guise of preventative medicine; and for performing oophorectomy (removal of ovaries) and hysterectomy operations on women without their consent. I am unrepentant about the conclusions I draw in this book and I urge all women to take to heart the very real risks they run when they come into contact with gynaecologists who recommend unnecessary hysterectomies.

This book presents the case against hysterectomy. However, I choose to begin with the case for hysterectomy to dispose of the few good reasons in support of it.

PART I

The Case for Hysterectomy

Statistical justification and contradictions

That there is an argument for hysterectomy is indisputable, although the number of cases where it is the correct therapy for women is less than 10 per cent of the actual number of operations – about 100,000 – performed each year.[1]

WOMB (UTERINE) CANCER

Hysterectomy involving the removal of the womb is obviously the only solution where cancer is proved to be present. Some gynaecologists remove the ovaries and cervix as well although it is debatable whether this is necessary if the cancer is confined to the womb. Cancer of the womb (uterus) has an incidence of 4,089 cases a year[2] from which three out of every 100,000 women die – 869 deaths per year.[3] The cancer affects the lining of the womb, the endometrium, and the cells become thickened in a condition called endometrial hyperplasia. This thickening of the endometrium, although benign in itself and present in both young women and those approaching the menopause, may turn from a hyper-stimulated condition into a pre-malignant one.[4] Cancer of the womb is treatable and there is a 70 per cent five-year survival rate[5] – that is 70 per cent survive for five years or more after treatment. Most cases of cancer of the womb occur in women who are over 60, the peak age being 65–69, with an incidence of 656 cases[6] recorded in 1990 (the most recent statisitics available).

Women of all ages must make certain that the operation they are being offered is not a prophylactic operation. Prophylactic operations, by their very name, are operations to prevent something happening which, in fact, may never occur. These operations are always unnecessary. Gynaecology is the only area of medicine where large numbers of patients are routinely subjected to preventative operations.

When endometrial hyperplasia is present samples of tissue are taken from the womb lining for analysis. This is usually done during a D&C (dilatation and curretage) operation, a minor operation which involves a day in hospital under a general anaesthetic. The womb is dilated and the lining is examined using a hysteroscope, a slender lightweight viewer which allows the gynaecologist to examine the lining of the womb. The womb lining is also 'scraped' and tissues removed for analysis, as well as small fibroid growths being removed. Smears from the lower womb and cervix can be obtained in the consulting room without an anaesthetic. The cells are then examined for abnormal, pre-cancerous or cancerous cells. Patients should insist on knowing the results of these tests to ensure that a prophylactic operation is not being prescribed.

OVARIAN CANCER

There is a case for oophorectomy where ovarian cancer is *proved* to be present – in fact it is vital for the patient. The immediate removal of the womb, ovaries, and fallopian tubes is the usual therapy for this condition, although it is disputable whether the womb and cervix need to be removed as well in all cases. Ovarian cancer is called the 'silent killer' because often it is not discovered until it reaches an advanced stage. It may well have spread to the surrounding organs, so removing the ovaries does not give protection from the disease. Some 5,700 new cases of ovarian cancer are detected each year[7], 70–80 per cent of which are fatal.[8] Fifteen out of 100,000 women[9] – 4,330 cases[10] – die of this disease every year and the survival rate over five years for those who are treated is only 20–30 per cent.[11] The percentage of cases which are found and treated is increasing, so the outcome for patients is improving if the cancer is caught in time. There is a greater incidence of ovarian cancer in women over the age of 60 with 66 per cent of the cancer occurring in older women. The incidence of ovarian cancer peaks between the ages of 65 and 74, with 1,566 cases recorded in 1990 (the most recent figures available).[12]

Ovarian cancer has proved difficult to diagnose but there are a number of tests which can help in detecting it if backed up with other evidence. There is a marker test for ovarian cancer, the CA-125 ultrasound immuno-assay test which is reckoned by London's Charing Cross Hospital Oncology Department, which monitors the test, to be about 70 per cent effective in tracing ovarian tumours. But it is just a marker test – that means it can only be used to help support a diagnosis of cancer if there is other more compelling evidence, such as a biopsy of tissues. Although modern ultrasound scans and tests help to support or disprove a diagnosis of cancer, they must be repeated over a period of time if there is any possibility of doubt about the diagnosis. In fact, a CA-125 test does not reveal anything significant about the progress of the cancer unless it is repeated. Patients must themselves insist that the tests are repeated, if there is any doubt about the diagnosis. Gynaecologists are well known for often prescribing a total hysterectomy – bilateral-salpingo oophorectomy (womb, ovaries and fallopian tubes removed), without repeating the test. Prophylactic oophorectomy (removing healthy ovaries) is the operation for which gynaecologists are most criticised by their patients. Women must make sure that any operation recommended is a necessary one because only then will they be able to come to terms with the physiological, psychological and emotional consequences.

CERVICAL CANCER

Cervical cancer is not now regarded with the same level of concern as it once was. Through a national screening programme the cancer cells can be detected at a very treatable stage. For most women who have this cancer, with conservative surgery, they will be able to retain their cervix and all of their reproductive organs. However, if the cancer is discovered at an advanced stage, it may already have spread to the womb and hysterectomy will be the only option. Cervical cancer has a 58 per cent survival rate over five years and affects 4,599 women a year.[13] Sixty-two per cent of cases occur in women under the age of 60; the peak age of incidence is 35 to 44,[14] with 1,095 cases annually[15]. However, most deaths from cervical cancer affect older women, those aged 70–74.[16] I can only assume from this that younger women are being treated successfully. Six out of 100,000 women[17] – 1,677 cases[18] – die from cervical cancer each year and 58 per cent of these women are over 60.[19] Cervical cancer is suggested through a smear which may show an early form of cell abnormality called cervical dysplasia.[20] A hysteroscopy may be used as well if the dysplasia is situated high up in the cervical canal close to the uterus. These cells may or may not become cancerous, but they do display microscopic changes. Most often found in young women between 25–35, the change from dysplasia to invasive carcinoma can be very rapid; and for this reason regular screening is advisable. Laser treatment to the cervix is the normal procedure where there is dysplasia and the cancerous cells are burnt away. Cryosurgery (low-temperature surgery) is sometimes used, and a conservative 'cone biopsy' is very likely to be used simply to remove tissues in which the carcinoma (cancerous growth) is situated.

PROLAPSED WOMB

Sometimes there is little alternative but to perform a hysterectomy for a prolapsed womb, and indeed, this may be the best solution for post-menopausal women. The ligaments which hold the womb in place stretch, particularly if a woman has had several large children. The loss of muscle tone which occurs after the menopause can result in the womb falling into, and sometimes through, the vagina. Hysterectomy is the most effective treatment for this condition, but it should only be considered as an option, along with the possibility of alternative treatments – supporting the prolapsed womb with a ring or re-suspending the womb and suturing or sewing it back into place. Younger women can have prolapsed wombs as well, due to damage caused by childbirth. For example, where the womb has been torn and badly repaired, it may prolapse.

For these conditions only – cancer and prolapse – is hysterectomy the appropriate treatment. For everything else – cysts, fibroids, endometriosis, heavy periods, painful periods and pelvic inflammatory disease – there are medical therapies and conservative surgical techniques which will preserve a woman's fertility and keep her organs intact.

STATISTICAL JUSTIFICATION

THE STATISTICS: WHAT DO THEY MEAN?

If present trends persist, one in five, (maybe one in four) women, is likely to have a hysterectomy by the time she is 60.[21] Each year 73,500 hysterectomies are performed on the National Health Service[22] and an unknown number, estimated as one to every three performed in the Health Service[23] are carried out privately, making a total of about 100,000 operations. Some 43 per cent of hysterectomies will also involve the removal of one or both ovaries; 60 per cent of those operations are performed on pre-menopausal women under the age of 49. According to a recent study, approximately 90 per cent of these will be unnecessary, and many women will suffer psychological and emotional trauma as a consequence.[24] Many will experience consequential damage caused by scar tissue ('adhesions') attached to bowel, intestines, bladder, pelvic wall or other organs, causing the patient excessive pain and distress. Some patients will have their bowel, bladder or other organs perforated or damaged during the operation, which may leave them permanently mutilated. And, sadly, 62 women, one in 1,600, die each year having this operation, presented as perfectly safe and routine. But safe and routine it is not – hysterectomy has a 47 per cent operative and post-operative risk factor, making it one of the riskiest gynaecological operations performed – something some gynaecologists omit to tell patients when prescribing the operation.

Medical reports demonstrate that the majority of problems women have with their wombs and ovaries are benign and non life-threatening – although they may cause discomfort. Why, then, is hysterectomy one of the most performed female operations (aside from abortion) in Britain, despite the fact that lung and heart disease are much more prevalent in the population? Gynaecologists justify themselves thus: if the whole of a woman's organs are removed, then no disease can develop in them. But this is a radical departure from how other areas of medicine operate – there the patient is treated for the condition he or she *actually has*, not a condition that they *might develop*. Widespread prophylactic surgery is done to counter the threat to a very small number of women. Gynaecologists admit, however, that even with overuse of hysterectomy and oopherectomy they have failed to reduce the number of deaths from ovarian cancer in the last thirty years.[25]

The only thoroughgoing study which links symptoms to diagnosis and recommended therapy was carried out in Dundee at the Ninewells Hospital in an exercise to assess the potential for new surgical techniques.[26] This study revealed that about 90 per cent of the women who were recommended to have a hysterectomy could have been treated more effectively and more cheaply with other therapies, including those offered by their GPs. Half of a sample of 100 women in the survey, interviewed in depth, expressed dissatisfaction with the recommendations and treatments they received.[27] In my opinion, gynaecologists would be providing a much better service to the nation and for their patients if they did nothing at all. The risk factor for a woman developing cancer in her ovaries is 3,800 for women over 25 and 2,500 in women over 55[28]; more than thirty times less risky than having an accident on the roads and more than eight times less risky than developing heart or lung disease.[29]

People naturally get very alarmed about cancer. However, it should be put in context. Cancer is present in 24.3 per cent of women and 28 per cent of men in the United Kingdom at some time in their lives.[30] Breast cancer is far more common than the cancers of the womb, cervix and ovaries put together[31]: 50 out of every 100,000 women die of breast cancer compared to 16 per 100,000 from all pelvic cancers.[32] Male prostate cancers are one and a half times as common as all cervical, ovarian and womb cancers,[33] claiming 35 per 100,000 men – twice the number of deaths from ovarian cancer.[34] Lung cancer is the most prevalent cancer in men – 95 fatalities per 100,000 men each year.[35] More common health risks are heart conditions – 340 cases per 100,000 of the population have hypertension, pulmonary and other heart diseases.[36] The risk to women of having cancer of either cervix, womb or ovaries is considerably lower than almost any health risk to men, and that includes vehicle accidents – there are 1275 vehicle accidents per 100,000 population annually.[37] So why are disproportionate public health resources allocated to women's health, and why has the number of hysterectomies increased by 25 per cent in the last fifteen years?[38] Why are half the hysterectomies performed on women under the age of 45[39] when the peak age of deaths from all the cancers of the cervix, womb and ovaries is 70–75?[40]

THE COST

A conservative estimate of the cost of unnecessary resources in gynaecology in the NHS is a staggering £500 million per year: employing gynaecologists and nurses, performing unnecessary operations, the use of buildings and hospitals, sickness benefit for patients, the costs of HRT prescriptions, post-operative treatments, and psychiatric after-care[41]. This vast sum could be better used for poorly-serviced areas of medicine where patients could really benefit from treatments and surgery.

PART 2

The Case Against Hysterectomy

Alternative surgical techniques and medical therapies

As I have said, the dreadful fact is that the vast majority of hysterectomies are performed for benign conditions which should never be treated with such unnecessary, harsh and costly surgery.

TWO TYPES OF HYSTERECTOMY

Basically, there are two hysterectomy operations: sub-total hysterectomy and total hysterectomy. The sub-total hysterectomy removes the womb but leaves the cervix in place. The cervix need never be removed unless the gynaecologist is *certain* that it is diseased, which can be easily and quickly ascertained through a cervical smear test or colposcopy (visual examination using a colposcope). The cervix is a part of the sexual apparatus which contributes to a woman's enjoyment of sex. For some, it is the trigger for orgasm and without a cervix a woman's pleasure may be severely reduced. She may not be able to enjoy sex to the full herself nor provide pleasure for her partner – a tragedy for both. Gynaecologists blithely tell their patients that the operation will not make any difference, but then they are in the 'business' of gynaecology and women's bodies are the essential requirement for the business.

An eminent gynaecologist has this to say about total hysterectomy: 'There are several ways of performing a hysterectomy, but the procedure usually used is called a "total hysterectomy". The operation removes the womb and cervix which is why it is called "total". Originally surgeons used to leave the cervix but this is no longer done because the cervix would remain a potential site for cancer.'

That there is patently little risk of developing cervical cancer, I have already established. With a nationwide cervical screening programme no woman should submit to this prejudice any longer, and should always demand to retain her cervix.

TWO METHODS OF PERFORMING HYSTERECTOMY

Of the two hysterectomy operations, vaginal hysterectomy and abdominal hysterectomy, the former is marketed more aggressively, although there is little to choose between them as both have a raft of negative effects. In the vaginal hysterectomy the gynaecologist removes the womb without cutting the abdomen. The severed tissues are drawn out through the vagina and the wound is sutured internally using a minute stitching gun. The advantage of this operation over abdominal hysterectomy is that there is no scar and the patient recovers much more quickly. All hysterectomies, except where women have large fibroid growths on the inside and on the outside of the womb, can be performed in this way. Many gynaecologists are not adequately trained in 'keyhole' surgery and there have been cases where patients have died because of incompetence with the technology.

The gynaecology business is dominated by middle-aged men with a 'traditional' attitude to their craft and they prefer to perform abdominal hysterectomies which present them with the opportunity of removing the ovaries as well. In an abdominal hysterectomy an eight-inch incision is made across the lower abdomen, just above the pubic hair line, to remove the womb through the abdominal wall. Abdominal hysterectomies have the disadvantage of severing nerves and therefore of removing sensation from the erogenous zone of the lower abdomen.

As I have said, it is becoming standard practice for gynaecologists to remove ovaries at the time of hysterectomy, especially in women over 45. Even worse, many women go into hospital to have lesser treatments only to discover on waking that a full hysterectomy and oophorectomy has been performed on them. Claire Merton, a medical journalist writing in *Vogue* magazine in November 1994 reported that: 'A gynaecologist privately told me in conversation, "If I had removed a person's ovaries I wouldn't tell them."'[1] Women recognise this as surgical assault, although there is no legal redress for victims of it, except to seek compensation through the civil courts. Some gynaecologists claim this is 'a preventative measure': they contend that the ovaries adhere to the pelvic wall and are therefore likely to become diseased if left in place.[2] No scientific study or evaluation, or proper medical trials, have been carried out to substantiate this claim.

One of the tragedies of gynaecology is that whims can be translated into surgical procedures without any kind of scrutiny or evaluation being carried out by an independent body and it is my belief that patients are being used as guinea pigs. Compare this with a drug company wanting to market a new drug: a drug has to go through a long process of testing and evaluation before it can be used, which may take many years. There is no such discipline for surgery. Gynaecologist A writes a short paper about his theory in a journal of

ALTERNATIVE SURGICAL TECHNIQUES

obstetrics and then he starts operating on his patients.
Gynaecologists B, C, and D sit in on the operation and if they like the look of it they will carry it out too. New surgical procedure becomes instituted entirely on the persuasion of individual doctors; a much safer practice would be to ensure that operations undergo scrutiny by an independent body.

The threat posed by prophylactic oopherectomy to women, especially to pre-menopausal women, is great:[3] they run the risk of developing osteoporosis, thrombosis and heart disease, as well as early macular degeneration of the eye, which can lead to blindness in later life.[4] And clinical depression and post-traumatic stress may blight their lives for many years. A computer model for prophylactic oophorectomy has been devised, inputting all the criteria relevant to ovarian cancer to acertain both the medical as well as the cost benefit.[5]

Some hysterectomies leave the patient with three-quarters of a vagina sewn up at the end. Some gynaecologists will cut the top of the vagina as well, even if cancer is not suspected, so that a woman is left with only three or three-and-a-half inches or less of vagina. With this a woman has not the equipment to enjoy sexual intercourse. It is a perfectly feasible operation to remove the womb without taking away the cervix and, in fact, is an easier operation to do, but this rarely happens. Some gynaecologists prefer to perform 'pelvic clearance' operations, and say that women's sex lives are improved. I have spoken to many women and have not come across one who would agree with this. And I know from my own experience that the reverse is the case.

Very few women are provided with sufficient information to give informed consent to this operation: doctors rarely present patients with brochures or publicity which represent anything other than the beneficial consequences of hysterectomy. How can a woman give informed consent if she is not told about the negative consequences as well? A gynaecologist conceded to me on a radio phone-in programme that hysterectomy was a 'brutal treatment'. Why then are so few women advised as to its effects or provided with help or advice before the operation and proper psychiatric care and counselling afterwards? Doctors have the opportunity to use conservative, non-invasive and reconstructive surgical therapies which have been developed in the United Kingdom, France and the United States.

Writing to a woman police constable, I said: 'To have your womb and ovaries taken away from you for no reason, or for little reason, has to be assault on a par with violent rape. It is a terrible and unwanted intrusion into a woman's most private and sensitive part of the body and, as with rape, the traumatic effects of it last for the rest of her life.'

THE RISKS AND VIABLE ALTERNATIVES

All surgery carries with it the risk of death or injury and patients should be aware of this. The risk of death or injury in gynaecological surgery is 1 in 1,200[6] and that risk should be compared with that of having a life-threatening gynaecological condition for which surgery is appropriate: 1 in 2,500. On this basis women should always opt *not* to have a hysterectomy unless convincing evidence of need has been presented to them.[7] There are perfectly good minimal, conservative surgical techniques: myomectomy, to remove fibroids, without removing the womb; myolysis to remove small fibroids through the vagina; treatments to the endometrium for heavy periods; conservative surgery to remove adhesions and endometrial laser surgery or diathermy (application of heat through high frequency electric currents using electrodes) for endometriosis. However, many gynaecologists do not want to perform these operations and continue to perform abdominal hysterectomy, an operation developed more than a hundred years ago.

ALTERNATIVE SURGICAL TECHNIQUES

FIBROIDS AND THEIR TREATMENTS

Thirty-seven per cent of abdominal hysterectomies are performed on women who have fibroids.[8] One alternative for these women is a myomectomy, which removes the fibroid growths from the womb but leaves the womb intact. This operation was the prescribed operation for pre-menopausal women with fibroids in the 1950s, but today it is claimed that it results in excessive bleeding of the womb post-operatively. I asked a leading gynaecologist who performs many myomectomies each year what he thought about this view and his response was that the heavy bleeding could be controlled with proper surgical care. A patient fought for three years to have the myomectomy she wanted to remove a large fibroid, instead of the hysterectomy she was offered, causing increasing irritation and annoyance to all the gynaecologists she encountered. Should women be subjected to this sort of pressure? Many women would not have such exceptional determination not to be mutilated.

Women are having hysterectomies for fibroids when the size of the fibroids and the imminence of the menopause does not justify them. Fibroids shrink after the onset of the menopause when the supply of oestrogen which feeds them and stimulates their growth reduces. These perfectly benign growths can cause no symptoms at all, occasionally they may result in heavy menstrual bleeding, but otherwise should be of no more concern. For most women over the age of 45 the best treatment for fibroids is to do nothing at all and let nature take its course.

But for a few women, surgical removal is necessary because the size and situation of the growths cause pressure on surrounding organs. The possibility of a myomectomy should be very good news for patients of all ages, but the skills available to perform this operation are in very short supply. I want all women to know that they have a right to demand it from their doctors. Nothing could guarantee change more than the prospect of women asserting what it is that they want.

Myomectomy is a more complicated procedure than hysterectomy. If the fibroid is large, then it will need to be shrunk, using drugs such as danazol or busorelin which stops the menstrual cycle and gives an artificial menopause. This treatment is undertaken a few months before the operation to give the drugs time to work. Fibroids are given a size-equivalent to that of a pregnant uterus. Generally speaking, fibroids do not need to be removed unless they become a problem to the functioning of surrounding organs, the bladder and bowel in particular, and this stage is usually estimated to be at 20-week pregnancy size. Smaller fibroids, however, may need to be removed depending on their type and position.

Fibroids grow on all parts of the uterus and are of three types. Those which grow on the exterior wall are called subserosal fibroids; intramural fibroids grow within the womb wall, and submucosal fibroids grow into the inside of the womb. Those which grow on a stalk, either subserosally or submucosally, are called pedunculated fibroids. Open myomectomy is principally used to remove fibroids from the womb, but subserosal and pedunculated subserosal fibroids are sometimes removed laparoscopically, using a laser through the abdominal wall. Hysteroscopic myomectomy is used mostly for submucosal fibroids and this is done through the vagina either with a scalpel, laser or electrodiathermy, which cut or 'shell out' the fibroids. Pedunculated fibroids are clamped and tied to remove the blood supply and then cut off. Recovery time for open myomectomy is similar to that for a total hysterectomy, three to four months.

Gynaecological operations are, generally speaking, delicate and it is known that the smaller hands of female gynaecologists produce less pain during clinical examinations and present less likelihood of damaging organs during surgery. But gynaecology is dominated by men, who, in my view, have been responsible for holding it back in the 19th century. Despite today's numerous treatments, the number of hysterectomies performed each year continues to climb.

Heavy menstrual bleeding and painful periods may be caused by fibroids, endometriosis or pelvic inflammatory disease. In many women, however, there is no cause found (dysfunctional internal bleeding). The birth control pill and associated drugs are the main medical treatments for these conditions. Hormone pills can be effective in reducing heavy bleeding. Danazol, a synthetic steroid hormone that inhibits pituitary gonadotrophins, is the principal drug for treating endometriosis and Provera for menorrhagia; high dose progesterone or the combined oral contraceptive pills, for example, Femodene, Marvelon, Minulet and Ovran, Microgynon-30. There is also a new treatment called buselerin which comes in the form of a nasal spray. For pelvic inflammatory disease (PID), caused by a variety of infective agents, some of which are sexually transmitted, the medical treatment is antibiotics based on an analysis of the cervical discharge. Chronic PID affects the fallopian tubes with scar-like tissue and causes infertility. PID is very likely to cause pain during intercourse (dyspareunia).

CONSERVATIVE SURGICAL TREATMENT

All of these conditions respond well to conservative surgical treatments. PID, for example, can be treated by removing the fallopian tubes along with the surrounding inflammatory tissue. For women with a menorrhagia, hysteroscopy will provide information on the state of the womb lining and allow a hysteroscopic myomectomy or a myolysis operation for the removal of small sub-mucous fibroids from the womb lining if this is appropriate. Conservative surgery to the endometrium, the cells lining the womb, significantly reduces or stops heavy menstruation. It is the endometrium which swells and stores blood to prepare the womb for a fertilised egg and, when conception has not taken place, sheds the blood in menstrual bleeding. But cells from the endometrium may escape into the pelvic area and attach themselves to ovaries, bladder, bowel and to the pelvic wall. Wherever endometrial cells are attached they will also bleed during menstruation in response to the endometrium, causing heavy periods and often considerable pain. This condition is called endometriosis when it is widespread throughout the pelvic area. These cells can be removed laparoscopically using optical fibre laser surgical instruments or diathermy. The cells are literally burnt away.

Endometrial ablation and endometrial resection are two other operations which help to correct problems associated with the endometrium. With endometrial ablation a powerful laser is directed into the womb via the vagina and ablates the lining permanently. The patient is usually given a hysteroscopy before the ablation and may be given Danazol to reduce the thickness of the endometrium. An instrument called a rectoscope is used to treat the endometrium. This is similar to the hysteroscope, but it has a wire loop instead of a laser and the instrument is used to 'shave' or cut into the lining. Ablation or resection may cause adenomyosis. This is a condition where endometrial cells have grown into the wall of the uterus.

By removing the endometrium, the patient will not have periods but the hormonal cycle will be maintained and the ovaries will continue to operate without any change. The lack of negative consequences makes this treatment far superior to hysterectomy. However, it is a more dangerous operation, as it is possible to puncture the womb and the surrounding organs. After an ablation, a woman has to be very careful about contraception, as becoming pregnant could be very dangerous. The complete recovery time from ablation and resection is less than a week and both operations are very effective. The physical recovery time from hysterectomy is 10–14 times longer. Hysterectomy has an effect on the ovaries if they are left, and a woman will experience her menopause within 2–12 years of the operation, on average about four years earlier than she would have done, because of the disturbance to the blood supply to the ovaries and to the hormonal system during the operation.

CYSTS

The formation of follicular cysts is a normal part of ovulation. But many women form benign cysts on their ovaries. If there are a number of cysts, the ovaries can become quite large and give cause for concern. The presence of cysts is very likely to result in a prescription for oophorectomy, on the unreasoned belief that all cysts are potentially cancerous. Two types of cyst are, in fact, very common: corpus luteum cysts and dermoid tumours. The corpus luteum cyst forms after ovulation and, instead of being absorbed, which is normal, after two weeks they may bleed. Dermoid tumours are very common in younger women and make up 10 per cent of all ovarian cysts; they are not dangerous in themselves but they can become very large and run the risk of rupturing. Both types of cyst can be removed, without removing the ovary. Cysts can either be drained, (aspirated), or can be removed laparoscopically. Unfortunately, many gynaecologists jump to the conclusion that a cyst is likely to be cancerous and recommend an unjustified total hysterectomy /oophorectomy operation.

The physiological, psychological and emotional effects of hysterectomy

Even patients who have wanted their hysterectomies and who have been properly prepared for the consequences admit that there are physiological and psychological effects which they have not been told about. As one woman said to me, 'It's not fair really, they (men) can keep their sex, we have to lose ours.'

This woman has been happy with her hysterectomy, but even she has gone through the process of mourning that some women experience on the loss of their womb. It is the loss of sex and fertility, youth and beauty which causes this grief. Men cannot experience it nor can they understand it; yet gynaecologists and GPs consistently deny that it exists, and they misinform their patients by telling them that there are no physiological or psychological consequences of hysterectomy. It is this misinformation which works against women. In consequence, there is inadequate counselling for women having hysterectomies and no counselling after the operation. Women and their families are left without help or support.

That there is a major barrier to understanding of the consequences of hysterectomy by gynaecologists and doctors is testified by Vikki Hufnagel, the pioneering American gynaecologist who has developed a new system of reconstructive surgery to preserve the female organs. I believe there are two reasons for this barrier.[1] First, straightforward prejudice, and second, medical papers and clinical trials. And both get in the way of studying individual patient response. Indeed, papers and trials simply reinforce the prejudices. A trial was carried out recently in Aberdeen which established that there was no difference in the occurrence of depression and emotional consequences between hysterectomy and endometrial ablation patients.[2] The basic flaw in this is that the 204 women who elected to go on the trial were not in any way a representative group. We know that there are some women, because of early psychological experiences, who *want* hysterectomies. But I believe that most would not. In my view the clinical trial, with its limited perspective, is an inappropriate method of obtaining subjective opinions from women about their operations. For this reason, I am glad that a survey of 10,000 women, selected by random sampling techniques, is being carried out by the Department of Public Health Epidemiology of London University.[3] These women will be asked their opinion of hysterectomy and its consequences for them. Large patient surveys, not clinical trials, are the key to understanding. The Mistletoe project, commissioned by the Royal College of Obstetricians and Gynaecologists in 1993 and carried out by St Mary's Hospital, Manchester, was a similar large sample survey of patients who have had conservative endoscopic surgery.

As long as there is no proper understanding of patient opinion, the process of misinformation is going to continue – taught to doctors in training, and to GPs and nurses. The solution is, I believe, in the hands of women. They can break the circle by telling their doctors that they want proper evidence for any recommended treatment, advice and counselling about the consequences of any operation and they can refuse to make any decision until these are supplied. Before my operation I asked my gynaecologist the following questions:

Question: *Will the operation take long?*

Gynaecologist: *About 45 minutes. The operation is not serious, not as serious as a gall bladder operation, for example.*

Comment: *Hysterectomy and oophorectomy are about the most serious operations that a woman can have.*

Question: *Will it affect sexual relations?*

Gynaecologist: *Not at all. You won't feel any different. I expect that you will be able to have sex again after about six weeks, but not before that.*

Comment: *Nonsense, women do not recover that quickly from abdominal hysterectomy or oophorectomy. Sex is the main casualty of hysterectomy as every women who has had one knows.*

Question: *How long will it take to recover?*

Gynaecologist: *The recovery time varies, but I would expect you to be feeling better after a few weeks.*

Comment: *It took me two years to make a complete physical, mental and psychological recovery from the operation. An experienced nurse told me that it is normal for recovery to take between one and a half to two years.*

Gynaecologists appear to hold the view that menstruation is such a nuisance to women that they will be absolutely delighted to be rid of it. Many women, though, look at it differently. Menstruation, however inconvenient, however painful and however heavy the bleeding is a monthly reminder of a woman's sexuality, femininity, youth and her ability to procreate, which she does not want to lose. This is central to a woman's psyche and dominates her physical, emotional and psychological functioning. No understanding of

PHYSIOLOGICAL AND EMOTIONAL EFFECTS

women can be achieved unless this is understood. Emotions and hormones and the menstrual cycle are intimately intertwined and even a woman who has no intention of ever having a child is governed by the hormonal soup which courses through her veins. That there is just a well of emptiness after hysterectomy/oophorectomy where womb and ovaries used to be I can testify to. Hormones have such a profound effect on us that it is difficult to know whether a reaction is physical or mental. That sex is profoundly important to individuals goes without saying. Gynaecologists, however, believe that giving oestrogen replacement will solve the problem after hysterectomy, and this is the basis of patient treatment. This treatment has no scientific foundation; on the contrary, there have been many papers and studies to show that the reverse is true.

PHYSIOLOGICAL EFFECTS

A woman's body goes through many physical changes after hysterectomy, and especially after hysterectomy/oophorectomy, including accelerated menopause and rapid ageing. What is certain is that women would not knowingly want to advance the ageing process. Evidently some women are not being informed this will happen; rather they are being told that HRT will in some way prevent this process – this is not true. It is common for a woman's body to change shape after hysterectomy as well, and she may experience vague aches and pains and continuous breast pain. The womb is the key pelvic organ because it holds all the other organs in place. With the womb removed there is a tendency for the bowel and bladder to prolapse into the open cavity leading to an eventual prolapse into the vagina. Also, most women tend to put on weight, particularly if HRT is prescribed; this may have to do with the natural process of storing oestrogen in body fat. This weight increase is also denied by some gynaecologists.

The operation affects mental functioning, causes short-term memory loss and alters emotional responses and perceptions as well, as all are governed by hormones. Even emotional experiences such as pleasure, joy, happiness, lose value, just as negative feelings do. A woman will be robotic and out of control. The trauma which her body has suffered causes hormonal imbalance and dramatic mood swings. The sex hormones – oestrogen, progesterone, testosterone – are metered from ovaries and adrenal glands in response to signals from the pituitary gland, to match the monthly cycle and prepare the womb to receive a fertilised egg. After hysterectomy, they cannot function in consort. HRT does not match the body's supply of oestrogen in quantity or timed response and this leaves a woman in a hormonal mess which takes a long time to re-balance through the adrenal glands.

Women are very prone to infection following a hysterectomy. The vagina is normally full of bacteria and in the course of the operation, even with the best preventative measures, there is a risk of infection spreading in the open pelvic area. One in every ten patients contracts an infection in hospital anyway, but because of the nature of hysterectomy the danger is higher[4]. Some infections, escherichia coli, for example, can travel back up into the kidney and cause permanent damage. Patients need to be watched very carefully in their recuperation period in the hospital, antibiotics taken, and temperature monitored for evidence of infection. Patients are especially liable to candida albicans infection ('thrush') and chlamydia if it was already present. Naturally, after a major operation the immune system is under stress and the body is prone to infection. There is some evidence that ovaries support the immune system – which is another reason for not allowing them to be removed unnecessarily.

After oophorectomy there is an immediate increase in the blood cholesterol level and the patient is more at risk from thrombosis and heart disease. Oestrogen protects the heart against disease. For women who are close to the menopause increased risk from heart disease will not be greater if they lose their ovaries. However, for women who have their ovaries removed in their twenties or thirties, or even forties, there is a risk. One woman who had her ovaries removed when she was 35 without oestrogen replacement died suddenly aged 65 from a pulmonary embolism. As no research has been carried out into the connection with early death from heart disease and strokes due to pre-menopausal hysterectomy and oophorectomy it is only possible to speculate that women are dying early because of these operations. Women who have been able to keep their organs beyond the menopause stand a much better chance of reducing their risk of heart disease, because ovaries continue to secrete small amounts of oestrogen for up to twelve years afterwards. This oestrogen also protects the bones from osteoporosis, and eyes from macula degeneration (which leads to blindness in old age).

Hysterectomy has a psychoendocrinological effect – in other words, hormones affect the psychological state of the patient. Large amounts of FSHs (Follicle Stimulating Hormone) are present immediately after the operation which gives the patient a 'high'.[5] Later, usually within six to twelve months, there is a dramatic drop in the FSH level which puts the patient into a sort of 'hormonal shock'. It is at this time that most women become depressed and their depression deepens with time. Women should be treated with SSRIs – serotonin inhibitors such as Prozac – to control the worst effects, but according to one study by Elizabeth Armstrong many GPs do not recognize depression and consequently do not treat it. Depression damages relationships and destroys any desire to participate in life. I found it impossible to do the simplest of things, I could not remember anything, and I did not sleep at night. My husband described this as 'being unstable' for many months. But my experience of it was more like being blank: I used to prowl round the house at night and ring the

Samaritans when I got desperate. I cannot recall much of my awful mental state now, but I know I did little during that time – I could not clean the house or do any of the essential things I needed to do. Even small household tasks became major projects which I could not contemplate and I am typical of many women who become severely ill through depression following hysterectomy.

PSYCHOLOGICAL AND EMOTIONAL CONSEQUENCES

Gynaecologists say that there are no psychological and emotional consequences of hysterectomy and that it is only women who were depressed before the operation who are depressed after, thus blaming women themselves. They say that the menopause does not cause depression either. Both of these claims are clung to by a male-dominated gynaecology profession at the expense of their patients. The experience of thousands of women from different walks of life would indicate that the contrary is true, but their opinions are never sought. Oophorectomy affects that part of the self which identifies with the feminine image.

Deprived of her identity, with both her body and mind affected, she is certain to be subject to depression. Some gynaecologists and doctors dismiss this as not worthy of consideration, but women suffer excruciating mental distress as a result of this operation. My general practitioner turned his head aside whenever I said I was depressed. I had to change my GP to get treatment for my debilitating depression which lasted for two years. I know many women whose lives have been ruined through depression, because they cannot cope with the effects of the operation.

Post-hysterectomy depression, if it were caused *only* by an unnecessary operation, could be explained by lost self-image. But it arises out of the powerlessness that women feel about their bodies and the treatments they receive at the hands of doctors. Gynaecology is the only branch of medicine where the doctor coerces the patient into having an operation. For example, one woman who was newly married and desperately wanting to have a child, woke up from an operation she expected to be a routine non-gynaecological treatment, only to discover that her ovaries had been taken from her without her consent. She suffered not only physical distress but also excruciating mental trauma which she is still experiencing years later. No one in the hospital would explain why this had been done to her, no one would admit that it was done wrongly, and no plausible reason was given to her GP either. The hospital doctors fell over themselves justifying their actions, instead of providing care for the patient. A woman in that situation then has to summon up the energy to sue the doctor and the hospital because there is no provision in statute law for action against a doctor – and this she has to do at a time when she is at an all-time physical and mental low.

According to one survey in the 1980s[6], 70 per cent of women who have hysterectomies experience depression, and 6 per cent require psychiatric treatment. I have spoken to many women, who, like me, suffered Post Traumatic Stress Syndrome, a deeply disturbed state of mind involving terrible, vivid flashbacks. In the face of all of this, I am constantly amazed by women's courage and endurance.

The effect of hysterectomy on sex and relationships

Sex and love are the prime motivators in life. You cannot read a novel, watch a film, listen to music, without being aware of the potent and powerful effect of passion, sex and love on human beings of all ages. To be a castrated woman is to be cast out from normal emotional feelings and attitudes so that you are unable to experience the most profoundly important part of what should be your life, and you become aware of your isolation from those feelings which, in turn, causes distress and depression.

The foremost sexual psychologist, the American Alfred Kinsey, who made a lifetime study of human sexual response, described in his book, *Sexual Behaviour in the Human Female*,[1] the function of the organs in sexual intercourse:

> *Many females, and perhaps the majority of them, find that when coitus involves deep vaginal penetrations, they secure a type of satisfaction which differs from that provided by the stimulation of the labia and the clitoris*

alone. In view of the evidence that the walls of the vagina are ordinarily insensitive, it is obvious that the satisfactions obtained from vaginal penetration must depend on some mechanism that lies outside the vaginal walls themselves ... The cervix has been defined by some of our subjects, as well as many who go to gynaecologists, as an area which must be stimulated by the penetrating male organ before they can achieve full and complete satisfaction in orgasm.

The American gynaecologist, Don Sloan, wrote in 1978[2]:

Perhaps one of the more subtle and effective myths of sexuality has been that there is 'better sex' without the uterus ... How convincing can we be in assuring our patients that their sexual responses will not be affected after hysterectomy? Indeed, now we are becoming increasingly knowledgeable in sexual anatomy and physiology, how sure are we that the uterine secretory function and mobility and the physiologic reactions during coitus with a partner or masturbation do not play a role in determining some degree of sexual pleasure.

Female sexual response then is dependent upon the presence of the cervix and the vagina – the very organs which gynaecologists tell us we will not miss if they are removed.[3] Female orgasm is not an optional extra for most women – indeed, it is what is most sought after in sex. Without orgasm neither man nor woman finds there is much point to sex, and this often becomes the focus of problems in relationships. Womb and ovaries govern female sexual desire. They define women as sexual beings and prescribe sex and sexual relations because it is the secretion of hormones which creates libido and sexual functioning. These secretions – principally testosterone – provide a woman with her 'drive' and energy; women who have had a hysterectomy are almost uniformly lacking in sparkle. Normal sexual arousal is created by stimulation and foreplay which causes the clitoris to lengthen and swell, the vagina to enlarge and mucus secretions to flow. The whole genital system becomes swollen with blood and the uterus (womb) begins to rise in preparation for intercourse. Breasts swell by as much as a quarter of their size and nipples become erect, increasing their length by as much as 1 centimetre and 0.5 centimetre in diameter.

Without a womb and cervix, and especially without ovaries, a woman ceases to be a sexual woman and she is reduced to the hormonal state of a pre-pubescent girl or a very old woman. Hormones control our physical and mental processes and without our organs none of the arousal responses works, either mentally or physically. The nipples will not become erect and no amount of stimulation of the clitoris will exact a response from the truncated vagina. Research carried out in the United States has revealed that all hysterectomy patients experience a high incidence of decreased or absent libido, whether or not their ovaries are retained, and that oestrogen replacement does not restore libido following hysterectomy, although it does counteract vaginal dryness and atrophy and reduces menopausal symptoms. In spite of this, general practitioners and gynaecologists continue to tell their patients that a hysterectomy will not affect their sex lives, will not change them, and that they will feel no different. Women should disregard these views because they are clearly untrue. I doubt there are many women who come through a hysterectomy without some post-operative sexual problems.

From other research studies carried out in the USA it is known that the most ardent supporters of hysterectomy among women are those who identify the womb as sinful or dirty or wicked.[4] Many of these women have been the victims of incest, rape, childhood sexual abuse or an unwanted pregnancy. These women are so vocal in support of hysterectomy that gynaecologists believe this to be the norm of feminine opinion.

Women are clearly faced with a dilemma if they *are* presented with true information about the consequences of hysterectomy: they alone must be able to decide whether to have this most serious operation, or not. If a woman's pain, or continuous debilitating condition, is so severe that a hysterectomy is the only reasonable solution after other lesser therapies have been tried, it may well be that she will feel so much better from the relief of pain that she is prepared to live with a subsequently less satisfactory sex life. What is certain for all hysterectomised women is that sex will not be improved by having a hysterectomy, as is often stated in books and magazine articles written by gynaecologists. Every woman I have spoken to tells me that they have little or no sex following a hysterectomy, so it is reasonable to conclude that a hysterectomy is the antidote to sex.

Many women, particularly oophorectomised women, experience extreme reactions following hysterectomy, such as not being able to bear to have their husband or partner touch them, or even to be able to feel comfortable speaking to a man. For a while I would even panic if alone in the same room as a man and consequently had to ensure that I would always see a woman doctor, accountant, solicitor, banker, and so on. I have often felt the desire to be completely on my own since my operation, without the responsibility or the love of my husband to help me, and feelings of this kind are obviously destructive to relationships.

Our sex hormones are vital to our physical, mental and emotional well-being. We are neutered, a different species and, like the cathedral castrati, an object of pity. Male gynaecologists, who can never be in a position to understand our grief, add insult to injury in telling us that we are neurotic to have these feelings. When we become psychologically distressed they tell us that we 'make ourselves ill' and are therefore not deserving of help. Their attitudes are callous when they should be kind and considerate.

I have received many letters from women testifying to the serious effect hysterectomy has on their sex lives, how their husbands and partners find them unsuitable sex partners after hysterectomy and how this contributes to the break-up of their relationships. One woman was married for many years to a man she still loves, but one year after her hysterectomy her sex life was 'non-existent'. 'I just couldn't seem to get on with my husband anymore – I just didn't feel a complete woman. I am depressed and I cry a lot.' This is the tragic story of many women.

The loss of womb and ovaries does in some way change women so that they are different people. Everything – intelligence, perceptions, outlook, energy levels, zest for life – is affected. A group of hysterectomised women who set up a self-help group cited 'lack of motivation' and 'loss of self-esteem' to be among the main effects experienced. Sex drive gives women the desire to look after themselves, to diet, to keep in shape, to dye their hair, to dress well. What many women experience after hysterectomy is that there is no motivation to do these things. Depression contributes to the process which becomes a vicious and self-destructive cycle. Somewhere in the middle of this is the husband or partner who is very often completely at a loss to understand what is happening to the woman once dearly loved and now increasingly estranged. Sex is the first thing to go in the relationship.

And, tragically, as she becomes more emotionally dependent, her partner becomes less so. The script for this scenario has been devised by the gynaecology business but the tragedy is being enacted in hundreds of homes all over country as you read this page.

It is obvious that hysterectomy affects marriages, relationships and family life, but husbands and partners are almost never involved in the decision-making or counselled in any way about the profound changes that will happen as a result of hysterectomy.

Ageing, the menopause, HRT and hysterectomy

There is almost no treatment, potion, cream, exercise or regime which women will not subscribe to to retain the blessedness of youth and the bounty of beauty. Our society demands it. Women are almost exclusively judged by their looks by men and, however many degrees or qualifications they have, their career progression and success depends on their suitability being judged almost entirely by men. Successful men do not want to be surrounded by women disparagingly regarded as 'past their sell-by date', so only those with youth or the appearance of youth, will do. It is precisely because women want to keep up with other or younger women that they seek help from gynaecologists. Menstrual flooding in the middle of a Board Meeting is no help to a woman climbing the ladder in middle life, neither is debilitating menstrual pain caused by endometriosis to a younger woman.

'Of course you will not feel any different after a hysterectomy,' said with such trained and cultivated assurance by a smiling male gynaecologist to a worried patient, is very comforting and plausible, however completely misleading and untrue. Women, especially if they have had children, are not bothered by the notion of losing their womb (after all it has served its purpose) if it means that they can carry on exactly as before, but without the problems of painful periods, heavy bleeding, tiredness, or anaemia. What women cannot bear to lose, though, is their youth and looks. If women were told that this went with the package, that in having a hysterectomy they would be opening a Pandora's Box and letting loose the menopause, rapid ageing and loss of sex drive, they would almost universally reject this option in favour of less drastic remedies. Just to prove this point, I tell the following story: A husband contacted me a short while ago about his wife, aged thirty-eight, due to have a hysterectomy in two weeks' time for fibroid growths described as being equivalent to a ten-week foetus in size. She was worried about having the operation and he was very concerned for her. When I spoke to the woman, however, she was sceptical about what I had to say. Surely the gynaecologist would not recommend an unnecessary operation? He must have a good reason? It was only when we got to talking about the effects of the operation that her attitude began to change. When I mentioned what hundreds of women I had spoken to have told me – namely that hysterectomy had aged them, and aged them visibly and rapidly, she immediately decided that she did not want to have the operation and told her husband to cancel it there and then.

THE MENOPAUSE

The menopause is talked about a lot, but is understood very little by women and doctors alike. A natural menopause is triggered by a declining number of eggs present in the ovaries. Nature provides every woman with about 400,000 eggs and an egg is released every month until she reaches the menopause. Women will still have some eggs at the onset of the menopause, so no one can accurately predict when it will occur and GPs always seek guidance from family history. The menopause is divided into three distinct periods: peri-menopausal, menopausal and the post-menopausal phases. Even for those few women whose path is relatively problem-free, menopause is what Germaine Greer calls a of 'rite of passage' with a number of effects – physical, spiritual, emotional and psychological.

We are accustomed to talking about the menopause as if it happens overnight, but nothing can be further from the truth, as the whole process can take as long as twenty years and each phase lasts for several years.[1] The peri-menopausal phase which may last as long as ten years before the menopause, is characterised by increasingly long and heavy periods irrespective of whether a woman has fibroids or not. My peri-menopausal phase started with a heavy menstrual flood on a business trip in 1982 and lasted until my hysterectomy in 1993. This heavy bleeding is quite normal and there is no reason to see a GP unless the effect is debilitating. The peri-menopause progresses towards the menopause with increasingly erratic menstruation in length, timing and heavyness. The dividing line between the peri-menopause and the menopause is not always obvious. A woman may go for many weeks or months without a period and then inexplicably they come back for a time. Feelings of dizziness, tiredness, thrush and recurrent bouts of cystitis are common at this time. The menopause begins with the cessation of the menses and menopausal symptoms of headaches, pins and needless, dizziness, hot/warm flushes, nightsweats, cystitis, feelings of weakness, sleeplessness, short-term memory loss, depression and dramatic mood swings increase with time. The menopause is a mirror-image of the onset of the menses, with all the problems that puberty brings. Menopausal women, like pubescent girls, feel that they are out of control of their bodies, something else has taken over – the effect of changing hormonal reactions.

Whilst puberty prepares girls for fertility, womanhood and motherhood, menopause prepares women for old age. The body has decided that she is too old to bear children, which brings with it feelings of rejection and depression. The skin changes, it becomes coarser and loses its bloom. Skin which has been plumped up gets thinner and dryer and wrinkles easily. Hair goes grey and becomes coarse and dry. Breast tissue changes its texture; it become less dense and so breasts sag. The menopause is often characterised by a continuous low-level depression. The short-term memory loss which women experience at this time contributes to depression because it feeds into loss of self-esteem resulting in a lack of self-confidence. Because society places such value on youth, it marginalises maturity, and menopausal women are most cruelly set aside from the mainstream of life. Menopausal women are most likely to be the first to feel the cold hand of redundancy.

Little is known about the function of the ovaries after the menopause, nor about the complex interaction of hormones secreted from the ovaries, womb, adrenal and pituitary glands, and how this affects the immune system and the functioning of the body as a whole. An eminent male gynaecologist whom I respect has even written that having a hysterectomy 'will not leave women feeling physically below par, prematurely old and depressed'. However, this view has no scientific evaluation, nor is it based on a comprehensive survey of patients' opinions. What gynaecologists are really saying is that *theoretically* this should not be the case based on their limited knowledge of the subject. Hysterectomy removes one, and often two elements, so two have to provide the function formerly supplied by four. It is neither logical nor possible that 4 minus 2 can add up to 4. Something is lost, and as the loss of ovaries is a massive trauma which dictates the passage of the body into a post-menopausal stage the ageing is so swift you can see it happening. I was always told how young I looked before I had my hysterectomy, and this was because, even at fifty-one, I was still ovulating, but two years after the operation I have visibly aged by five years. At fifty-one a woman is post-menopausal full stop, in spite of scientific evidence that women are entering the menopause at a much later date. It is not unknown for women to retain their fertility until their late fifties and only to be in the post-menopausal phase in their sixties. The cause is not understood, but it seems reasonable to suppose that it has something to do with better nutrition and fewer pregnancies. And women who do not have children, generally speaking, experience a later menopause.

Gynaecologists hold views about younger women which do not square with current knowledge and understanding. A woman of thirty-five is judged to be past childbearing, according to gynaecologists, and therefore a candidate for hysterectomy and oophorectomy. But statistical surveys of modern life reveal that more and more career-minded and working women are starting their families in their thirties.[2] Given the opportunity, gynaecologists will take out the wombs and ovaries of women in their late twenties and thirties and pack them off to an early menopause with no compunction whatsoever. In my opinion, no woman should be menopausal at so young an age unless it is dictated by proven cancer of the womb or ovaries. These women are then subjected to early menopause and ageing, with serious consequences for the health of their heart and bones.

HORMONE REPLACEMENT THERAPY (HRT)

Of course, the justification for gynaecological interference is HRT, Hormone Replacement Therapy; the oestrogen supply from the ovaries, removed from the body by oophorectomy, can theoretically be replaced artificially. Gynaecologists have fallen overboard for this notion – it is their new fad. However, the history of British medicine is littered with adherences of this kind, but history also reveals that much vaunted 'miracle drugs' are often found to be dangerous in the long run. HRT is no exception. Dr Ellen Grant, author of *Sexual Chemistry*,[3] a book about hormones, has said that HRT is not safe for long-term use, that there is a considerably increased risk of patients developing breast cancer. Even the gynaecologist John Studd, an enthusiastic advocate of HRT, has said that 'HRT increases the risk of breast cancer in women by 20–30 per cent over 8–10 years'.[4] For women who have their organs intact such advice gives them the opportunity to use it or not to use it. But for women who do not have their ovaries, they have no choice because if they do not take HRT they are at risk of developing osteoporosis which is a dreadful prospect. For women whose ovaries are removed in their twenties and thirties there is no alternative – they are going to be dependent for many years, possibly twenty or more, on a drug which is untried and possibly unsafe for long-term use.

The drug companies and their supporters, the independent charity The Amarant Trust, gynaecologists, women GPs and even some women politicians, have formed a powerful lobby for HRT. Only the positive benefits are marketed to women through a sophisticated and 'no money spared' public relations campaign. Women are not being won over, however, and only one woman in ten who is eligible for HRT actually takes it, and most who do give it up within one year.[5] Some women are not suited to HRT; they suffer from nausea, headaches and a variety of aches and pains; and for them it is just not worth it. But for many others it does provide help. The haggard appearance of women who have had hysterectomies or oopherectomies is alleviated by HRT because oestrogen has the effect of plumping up skin cells which gives the skin a smoother appearance and muscular strength is improved. HRT also has a good track record in reducing joint pains as well as alleviating short-term memory loss. It is interesting that HRT is now being used to prevent and relieve the symptoms of Alzheimer's disease which causes premature senility. We know that HRT can never replace the quality and quantity of oestrogen secreted from our own healthy ovaries, but the connection with Alzheimer's does indicate to me that the potential for premature senility is being added to the list of negative effects caused by prophylactic oophorectomy.

Case studies

The eight case studies described here are true, although to protect the women concerned I have changed some of the names and used first names only throughout the text.

CHRISTINE

Christine, then aged forty-one, had experienced twenty years of painful periods due to endometriosis. In 1992 she went to see a local gynaecologist privately and was referred for a trans-vaginal scan. The scan showed a large cyst on the right ovary and a smaller crystallised cyst on the left ovary. She saw a consultant who recommended an immediate operation to remove her right ovary and part of her left, but her womb, which was healthy although retroverted and 'stuck' to the abdomen by endometriosis, would be left. The operation was carried out privately. She was recommended to take testosterone after the operation to stop the onset of menstruation, as well as 'to tidy up' the endometriosis which was found to be present around the womb ligaments. A 200mg dose, which was doubled by her GP, gave her dreadful side effects – headaches, confusion, weight gain (she put on a stone) – so she stopped the treatment after six months. The drugs had failed to stop menstruation anyway. In 1995 a scan revealed that she had developed a cyst on the left ovary as well as on the womb. She was told that there was no option now but to have a hysterectomy and oophorectomy. The previous operation had been traumatic for her and she had been off work for six months, so she was adamant that she did not want another operation. She asked for a laparoscopy and a biopsy of the cyst but was refused on the grounds 'that if cancer was present the cells would spread'. She went to another consultant and asked her if the cyst could be aspirated and was told that the cyst could return. She had a negative CA-125 reading but still the gynaecologist would not consider anything but radical surgery. Christine was desperate when she came to me. I had made contact with one of the best gynaecologists in the country and had an arrangement with him that he would see any woman, like Christine, who could not get the treatment she wanted from her own gynaecologist. She went to see him and he aspirated and analysed her cyst in the consulting room. She wrote to me to say, 'It was the best Christmas present. He felt it was totally unnecessary to do a hysterectomy/oophorectomy and the weight was taken off me then and there and was absolutely fantastic.'

CLARE

Clare, aged fifty-one, had suffered from heavy periods for seven years when she first consulted her GP in 1987 and was prescribed Dicynene. But the tablets were only marginally helpful, so a year later she was referred to a gynaecologist. Clare had a D&C which helped, but after a while the periods returned to their pre-D&C level. She was then prescribed Ponstan Forte which she took with Dicynene which resulted in heavy night-time flooding. In 1991 she learned that a gynaecologist who is one of a group promoting keyhole surgery, was recruiting patients to try out a new technique, TCRE (transcervical resection of the endometrium), and Clare went to her GP to volunteer herself for the trial. She needed to have a hysteroscopy before she could be accepted on the trial and was referred to another London hospital in July 1991. In the consultation, Clare explained to the registrar that she had not sought help before because she did not want a hysterectomy. Clare had a hysteroscopy and D&C in January 1992 and was finally admitted for the TCRE in April 1992. Clare saw her gynaecologist and he told her in front of a group of students that 'she was a suitable candidate for TCRE'. When Clare came round from the operation she was aware that she had a pain across her abdomen and a doctor was telling her that the gynaecologist 'had carried out a hysterectomy as that was the best thing'. She expressed her anger and outrage. She was told later that not only her womb had been removed but both ovaries as well. She said that she would sue him but was told that as she had signed the consent form, she had given her consent to the operation. The gynaecologist said he had found a 'swelling', (which Clare discovered later was a fiction), so he had decided to proceed with the full hysterectomy/oophorectomy operation without even attempting the operation for which he had been given consent. Clare was so traumatised by her experience that she felt she could not bear to stay in the hospital a minute longer. She discharged herself and, with the help of friends, neighbours and her General Practice Nurse, she recovered physically from the operation but psychological recovery has taken much longer and she still has fits of depression. Clare questioned the gynaecologist later about his decision. He said that he discovered adenomyosis and in any case that 'it was up to him to decide what treatment a patient had', not the patient.

DIANA

Diana, aged fifty-one, had experienced a twenty-one day period and, because she had a D&C five years earlier, decided to go to the doctor. The GP felt the abdomen and said 'you have fibroids' and sent her to a gynaecologist at the local hospital. In 1993 she saw a woman gynaecologist at her local hospital and Diana showed her the five-year record of her periods she had kept – information about the frequency and heavyness of her periods. Two weeks later the gynaecologist said that she would not do a hysterectomy because Diana was peri-menopausal. She was sent for a scan and the scan was repeated four weeks later. In her place at the next consultation was a male gynaecologist. Straight away he started talking about cancer and a hysterectomy/oophorectomy operation because they had found an ovarian cyst on her left ovary. Diana was very upset. There had been no question of cancer in her discussion with the previous gynaecologist. He said that he had put her name on the waiting list for an operation, but Diana refused, saying that she was not convinced it was necessary. He wrote to her and said that cancer could not be ruled out, that it was normal practice to recommend total hysterectomy/oophorectomy operations, and that even if they agreed to do a laparoscopy then they would very likely 'proceed to a full hysterectomy/oophorectomy operation without consulting the patient'. Diana was furious and wrote back saying, 'You can just take my name off the list'. For two weeks the GP practice rang her every day asking her to make an appointment to see the GP, which she declined. Eventually the GP rang her and threatened to strike her off his list if she did not have the operation. Her resolve was weakened and she agreed to see the consultant gynaecologist. The consultant blatantly lied to her and played up the cancer risk so alarmingly that she agreed to the operation which was arranged in ten days time. She discovered one year after the operation that all she had was a dermoid ovarian cyst and that the operation had been unnecessary.

Diana suffered serious trauma as a consequence. It took her five months to recover physically and two and a half years to recover psychologically and emotionally.

FRANCES

Frances, aged forty-seven, went to see her GP in the summer of 1992 as she had an unexpected bleed between periods. The GP found that she had a uterine polyp and she was referred to a private gynaecologist. The gynaecologist removed the polyp during the consultation but said that he could feel a large cyst. He said that a scan should be done and the cyst removed. Frances agreed to the operation which was to be carried out in a local private hospital. When she woke after the operation she was very weak and uncomfortable and asked the nurse if this was normal. The nurse replied that after a hysterectomy this was to be expected. Frances responded that she had not had a hysterectomy but was assured that she had. It was later confirmed by the gynaecologist that a complete hysterectomy – what he called 'pelvic clearance' – removal of ovaries, womb, fallopian tubes and cervix had been performed on her. Frances was very shocked by the news but, weakened by the operation, was resigned to the situation. She was distressed because she had not been prepared for such drastic surgery; in fact, she had booked a holiday in France immediately after the operation and she had been unaware that cancer had been suspected. She discovered later that the cyst, although unusual, was not malignant. She suffered five months of disturbed sleep, anger and frustration and decided to write to the gynaecologist for a detailed account and explanation as to why he had performed such a serious operation without consent. He replied that the operation was standard treatment for cancer, and that she was mistaken if she had thought at any time he would just be removing the cyst. From her medical notes Frances learned that there had been no mention of cancer either before or after the operation. With a solicitor recommended by Action for Victims of Medical Negligence (AVMA) she sued the gynaecologist for negligence and trespass and in 1995 received a five-figure sum in an out-of-court settlement. Frances has since discovered that her cyst was performing an unusual function for her by collecting thyroid, because her thyroid gland was not functioning properly. She is now being treated for thyroid deficiency.

GLORIA

Gloria, aged forty-four, suffered from heavy and painful periods and had become quite anaemic. Her GP, without doing any investigations or attempting to treat her himself, said, 'you have BUPA, don't you – I'll refer you to a gynaecologist.' The gynaecologist gave her a brief examination and recommended a vaginal hysterectomy. He said that she would be 'better off without it', referring to her womb as 'a redundant organ'. He promised her that she would be back at work in six weeks and that she would have no scars. She agreed to have the operation for fibroids and adenomyosis. The operation went well and Gloria appeared to be recovering well until ten days later she was bent double with a searing pain in her abdomen and vagina. For six weeks she lived in agony and was put through a series of excruciating tests. The gynaecologist and a surgeon carried out a laparoscopy and found bowel adhesions to the vaginal vault wound. The adhesions had to be severed by a laparotomy (cutting the abdomen), so she had a scar after all. She continued in pain and discomfort for many months, and the gynaecologist became very intolerant of her. Instead of six weeks, she was away from her job for four and a half months. After a few years she felt better but five years later Gloria is again suffering from similar pains. She has yet again had to have tests to find out the cause and this time has had a laparoscopy and gastroscopy and she now awaits further tests and consultations. The laparoscopy

revealed further bowel adhesions but the surgeon is unwilling
to operate 'as they will only come back'; the gastroscopy was
inconclusive. She no longer has medical insurance and at the present
time she has been in pain for a year. Gloria wrote to me and said, 'It
could be debated as to whether my hysterectomy was necessary or
not. What I do feel strongly about is the fact that I was only told of
the best possible scenario. I would rather have put up with my bad
periods and taken my chances than gone through all the dreadful
things which have resulted from the hysterectomy.'

PAMELA ✳

Pamela, aged forty-one, was suffering from heavy periods. So in
the spring of 1990 she went to see her GP who, without giving her an
examination, said she could have a hysterectomy if her periods got
heavier. Pamela was a virgin and horrified at the idea of such drastic
surgery. She kept away from the doctor, but she began to show signs
of anaemia. She went back to her GP and asked for an iron test. The
test showed a haemoglobin level of 9 which meant that she was quite
anaemic (World Health Organisation definition of anaemia is a
haemoglobin level of less than 11). Pamela was referred to a woman
consultant gynaecologist at her local hospital and was told that she
had a 'large mass' which could be fibroids or an ovarian cyst and
the consultant could do a hysterectomy, or remove the ovary, or
everything ... ' She was sent for an ultrasound scan which revealed
a large fibroid in her womb, and a further blood test which revealed
a reduced haemoglobin level of 8.8. Pamela was completely against
having a hysterectomy, and having read up on the subject asked for
a myomectomy. She was asked to come back to see the gynaecologist,
but instead of the woman there was a male gynaecologist who tried
to pressure her into having a hysterectomy. She refused and,
distressed, cried all the way home. She was described as being
'a rather difficult lady' in the hospital records. She changed her GP

and in a letter described how traumatised she was by the visit to the hospital. She had lost a stone in weight and had become very nervous and weepy. Pamela had been treating herself with iron since her last blood test and the level was now normal but her fibroid had grown. Earlier she had contacted the College of Obstetricians and Gynaecologists and was surprised to be told that myomectomy was a 'frequently performed operation' and that her letter had been passed on to a Professor of Gynaecology in the north of England. She saw the professor in July 1993 and finally acquired a proper diagnosis of her condition. In March 1994 she was given 4 Zoladex injections to shrink the fibroid in preparation for the myomectomy operation. The fibroid that was removed weighed 530 grammes and was about 400 cubic centimetres in size. Pamela estimated that the fibroid had been about 1200 cubic centimetres at its largest. She recovered well from the operation and has suffered no ill effects.

SARAH

Sarah was thirty-nine when she began to suffer low backache and sciatic pain down her left leg but in spite of seeing her GP no effective treatment was supplied. Typically, the GP ascribed the problem to her womb and she was referred to a gynaecologist at her local private hospital. The gynaecologist reported that she had painful and heavy periods, pain on intercourse, stress incontinence and low backache and he advised her to have a hysterectomy saying that, 'There is no doubt that all your symptoms can be referred to the fact that you have a bulky retroverted uterus. You will be completely cured once the uterus has been removed.' The gynaecologist carried out a total abdominal hysterectomy and appendectomy but the tubes and ovaries were left. The operation did not rid her of the pain as promised; in fact, she was in a worse condition and had a new problem, depression. One year after the hysterectomy and still in pain she was referred to a consultant neurologist who found a lumbar disc protrusion and she was recommended to have surgery to her spine. At this time, because of the agonising pain she was suffering, she had referrals to see an orthopaedic specialist, a psychiatrist and the local pain clinic. She was convinced the problems started with her hysterectomy, so she was seen by another consultant who confirmed that the disc injury was the cause of the pain, that it was not associated with her womb and the hysterectomy was unnecessary. Sarah had a operation on her lumbar and sacrum spine but she was still in pain. She went back into hospital for a laparoscopy where it was discovered that the left ovary was bound down to the vaginal vault with adhesions and she had multiple cysts on the ovary. So the ovary was removed in a third operation. Sarah was still in pain so a year later she went back into another hospital but the neurologist said little could be done for her as the spinal problem had been left for too long. She has been in constant pain ever since. She is still very distressed; the prescription of an unnecessary operation has caused her such post-operative trauma and pain that she has had to give up her job as a teacher. Having the hysterectomy exaggerated the problem she already had with her spine and prevented the proper diagnosis of the problem disc, which with earlier treatment, could have been cured.

SHEILA

Sheila, aged thirty-nine, was prescribed a hysterectomy in 1993 when a fibroid was found in her womb. She and her husband had planned to have another child. They wanted a girl to complete their family of two boys, but they were told that with the fibroid this would not be possible and she was recommended a hysterectomy. Sheila was assured 'that hysterectomy was a common procedure, one that was performed daily in scores of hospitals all over the country' and by 1995 she had agreed to an abdominal hysterectomy. Her husband was not quite so happy about the hospital. He first became alarmed about her condition on the day of the operation because she had not returned from the recovery room until more than eight hours after she had gone into the theatre and she was in a semi-conscious state and very sick. On the day after the operation she was still drowsy, her pulse was weak, and a doctor was called. He did not arrive until two hours later; he did not do a proper examination and only prescribed Antacid. Both Sheila and her husband tried to summon help but no one seemed to want to pay any attention. If her blood pressure and pulse had been taken then it is likely that her condition would have been diagnosed. She was in awful pain and was prescribing herself large doses of morphine from the patient-controlled analgesia machine. The doctor returned to Sheila shortly after his first visit and by this time realised that something was wrong and a resuscitation team was called in, but it was too late. An artery had been punctured in the operation and Sheila bled to death. Her husband was alarmed by her condition from the beginning and had told both nurses and doctors that she was not well but his concerns were brushed aside. At the coroner's investigation an open verdict was delivered because key hospital records which would have attributed blame were missing. The coroner described the loss of the documents as 'sinister'.

GPs and gynaecologists – the National Health Service and private medicine

Reading the catalogue of ignorance, incompetence and brutality described in the case studies you would be forgiven if you came to the conclusion that there are no competent doctors and gynaecologists. Let me say that this is definitely not the case. There are good and very good gynaecologists and GPs who are delivering a caring, concerned and conservative service to patients, but finding these decent practitioners is difficult. Most GPs are not concerned about who are good and who are bad consultants, so patients have to find this out for themselves. Increasingly, women from all walks of life are coming to me in a very worried state about diagnoses given to them by their gynaecologists. General practitioners should be providing referrals for a second opinion but because they fail to do this a less than adequate service is being provided.

GPs AND GYNAECOLOGISTS

Blame for the situation in gynaecology must then be laid at the feet of general practitioners as well as gynaecologists. No one expects GPs to be gynaecological experts but patients do have a right to expect them to know enough to specify which treatment is appropriate to their condition, and to explain in simple but unpatronising language what might be wrong with them, what treatments are available, as well as the consequences of that treatment. The fact that this is done in only a minority of cases is an indictment of general practice as a profession. There can be no epithet too strong to describe this failure when it results in unnecessary surgery.

The following stories illustrate the depth of the lack of interest and ignorance displayed by GPs: A GP at the time told me with absolute assurance that 'women do not suffer from depression at the menopause. Depression is caused by other things like children leaving home.' It was a trite and dismissive statement guaranteed to turn any woman with depressive problems away from the surgery. A study carried out in 1995 confirmed the poor diagnosis and treatment of depression by general practitioners.[1]

A patient went to see an established, middle-aged woman GP in a Well Woman clinic. In the course of the consultation the GP told the patient that the ovaries cease to function after the menopause so she was better off without them. This patient had read up on the subject, and she argued with the doctor that ovaries continued to secrete hormones, including declining amounts of oestrogen after the menopause. The 'specialist' GP would not concede this until she was presented with incontrovertible evidence and had to admit that the patient knew more about the subject than she did.

Medicine is one of the few areas of employment which offers a job for life. Doctors only have to do something which offends their profession to be dismissed. Standards of acceptable conduct are set at a very low level with only professional misdemeanour and sexual misconduct attracting penalties. As doctors do not operate under any published and accountable professional code of practice they are, in effect, able to do whatever they like to patients, and incompetence is rewarded by transfer or promotion to another hospital, so the nuisance is swept under the carpet. Publicly exposed and incompetent consultant gynaecologists, however, are rarely reproved by their hospitals; in every case I have monitored they have kept their jobs and their privileges. NHS hospital administrators do not like incompetence because it attracts medical negligence claims which, if successful, have to be paid out of NHS funding. There is no pressure to provide conservative surgery, nor to ensure that doctors, surgeons and gynaecologists present acceptable attitudes towards their patients and are competent to perform their duties. This view was expressed forcefully by a former NHS Trust chairman who said that 'too little is being done to curb bad medical practice and Dr Dead Wood whose incompetence kills'.[2]

THE NATIONAL HEALTH SERVICE AND PRIVATE MEDICINE

The effective privatisation of the NHS which the government has justified as 'creating an internal market for services' through the 'reforms' of the then Secretary of State for Health, Virginia Bottomley, has contributed to the worsening situation for gynaecology patients as well as to escalating costs for gynaecological treatment in the NHS. A 'market forces' approach allows doctors to rig the market and put pressure on the suppliers (GPs) to provide more units (patients). It also encourages the processing units (hospitals) to 'polish the figures' for the 'management' (the government). In the 'market forces' medical economy, treating every patient as an individual and spending time on a number of tests to provide a proper diagnosis, giving more than one treatment, offering conservative surgery – all of this runs counter to the new factory ethos. Caring and conservative methods have been thrown out the window. Standardised industrial throughput methodology (which incidentally has now become an outdated concept in industry), is the rule, and thus only a limited number of standard treatments are provided for patients. It does not matter whether the patient, now denoted only by their number and not their name, from an appraisal of symptoms *needs* a hysterectomy, she is prescribed one because that is all that's on offer. She will then be stacked on the conveyor belt to wait her turn along with all the other 'operative units'. Hundreds of NHS 'factory' administrators and accountants have crawled over every action in the hospital 'factory' so that they are able to allocate a cost down to the last penny for every stage of the unit being 'processed'. So many women have described to me that they have been told by the 'reformed' NHS that they have got to have a hysterectomy they do not want 'or continue to suffer'.

Hospitals, which used to be places of diagnosis, treatment, caring and healing have been turned into 'surgical factories' with the throughput of bodies a much more important criteria than the level of health care delivered to the patient. In fact, an NHS Trust manager has said that patients come only third in the list of responsibilities that a doctor has: his first duty is to be loyal to his organisation, his second to himself.[3] GPs, who used to be patient-centred and caring professionals have been turned into accountants, rationing the time they spend with patients and resisting protracted treatments and costly actions so that their GP practice can make a profit. I was told by one GP that she could not give me more than one minute to discuss a matter that was unscheduled, even though it was important to me, because she could not claim for that minute and the practice would lose the revenue. The average consulting time is seven minutes. In seven minutes a GP is supposed to talk to the patient, examine them and form a correct diagnosis for treatment. It is not surprising then that so much goes wrong: it is a system designed for failure. Most GPs dispense with the talk and examination and send the patient straightaway to a gynaecologist, tapping in the patient number on their computer as a 'completed transaction'. A record is maintained against the quota of hysterectomy patients they are required to send to the hospital. And then they wash their hands of them – after all, the patients have been packed off to the factory to be processed from peas in a pod to peas in a tin and the GPs have performed their role.

There is a deep disquiet in the medical profession about the current state of the NHS and doctors and consultants have spoken out publicly against a system which places restrictions on their ability to provide patient-centred services. The old 'unreformed' NHS was in the words of one doctor, Dr Charles Clarke, 'very cheap, effective and much-loved' and this has given way to 'an explosion of bureaucracy and totalitarian silence'.[4] No one in medicine, least of all patients, is allowed to criticise the system. Doctors have always created cabals against their patients through their chauvinistic support of their fellow doctors. But now this old order has been overlaid with a new even more sinister regime which rations healthcare on cost reasons alone, and encourages and supports an explosion of hysterectomies against the wishes and good sense of women. Rather than achieving efficiency and cutting costs, which was the intention of the reforms, the reverse effect has been achieved and millions of pounds wasted. There is no mechanism to stop it. In the past, before GP fundholding and purchasing contracts with individual hospitals, GPs could send patients for second opinions to accredited experts. Patients today have no access to a second opinion except to purchase it privately, because GPs are under no obligation to provide a second opinion except from the hospital with which they have a contract. This effectively means that no second opinion is available because in a market economy no hospital is going to turn away the prospect of 'business'. And the situation is worsening as more GP fundholding practices acquire total purchasing power.

The NHS is used as a shopfront for private medicine. Women who come through the NHS door may well go out the door marked 'Private' so for some gynaecologists it is customary to have a few unnecessary operations stacked up to ensure a continuous supply. Dr Thomas Stuttaford wrote in *The Times* (10 October 1995) that among educated (graduate) women fewer hysterectomies were performed than among other women. Better educated women, it would appear, require more convincing that the operation is necessary than other women and are more likely to have it performed privately. However, even these women are not immune to persuasion and exaggeration, and the fear induced by the constant repetition of the word 'cancer'. And, of course, there is the prospect of personal financial gain for the gynaecologist. Consultant gynaecologists earn a very good living, the most aggressive of them making in excess of £150,000 a year, of which £70,000 is received from their NHS consultancy. In the USA, where gynaecology claimed the wombs of one out of every three women by the age of 70, the number of hysterectomies performed was proved to relate directly to the number of gynaecologists.[5] It has only been with the advent of protest from the women's movement that this regime has fallen.

Women should be warned and wary of private medicine for gynaecological operations. Some women have died in emergency situations in private hospitals because the hospitals were not equipped to deal with them. Nor do private health insurers vet the operations which are recommended to patients. If the gynaecologist decides to do something which was not agreed with the insurers in advance, the patient could end up having to pay, not only for the unscheduled operation, but for all subsequent treatment.

8

Seeking redress:
the NHS complaints system
and civil action in the courts

No woman expects to end up going to the police to cite her
gynaecologist for assault, or to sue her gynaecologist or hospital
for medical negligence as a result of what is described as a 'routine'
operation. But the fact is that this is what an increasing number of
women are doing, and gynaecologists who have always got away with
cavalier behaviour towards their patients in the past, are shocked by
this redress.

Gynaecology as a branch of medicine is attractive to a certain
type of man: a man who likes to be in control and in power. (And, of
course, most women are overly respectful to doctors.) When you add
arrogance, vanity and acquisitiveness to this profile it produces an
amalgam for trouble. I strongly believe that it is the psychological
make-up of these individuals, coupled with inadequate training
and education, which causes such professional malaise and the
same skill in the hands of more caring individuals produces very
different results.

✳ Sixty per cent of the complaints against doctors received by the General Medical Council, the doctors' disciplinary body, and one-third of all medical litigations are against gynaecologists – more complaints than in any other area of medicine. And these complaints are beginning to be heard: a gynaecologist has already been struck off the medical register for removing an ovary without consent and there are more in the pipeline. Woman are also winning actions in the civil courts although compensation for the loss of womb and ovaries and possible later ill health is still set at a lamentably low level – about £30,000. By comparison, a middle-aged man whose teeth were drilled unnecessarily by an unscrupulous dentist won his claim for £150,000 for a 'lifetime of dental work'. It appears that little value is placed on women and women's bodies. A woman was given a miserly £2,000 compensation for the loss of her womb, which the gynaecologist admitted he could have saved, and the family of a young single woman who died through medical incompetence at the hands of a gynaecologist received a paltry £5,000 compensation for her life. At a gathering of gynaecologists, rosy with port and after-dinner speeches, a gynaecologist announced with great mirth to his male colleagues that 'of course a woman's sexual organs are worth nothing – a man's are priceless'.

In an egalitarian age, how can women's lives be valued so low, when men's are valued so high? How can parts of a woman's body be given a value so much lower than the equivalent parts of a man's body? The truth is that compensation for parts of the body are decided jointly by the legal and medical professions, and it is therefore not surprising that gynaecology with its nineteenth-century mentality provides nineteenth-century levels of compensation for litigants. Specifying realistic levels of compensation would be a definite disincentive to those who are 'scalpel happy'; compensation has remained low and will stay low as long as those people remain in charge of their profession.

THE CASE AGAINST HYSTERECTOMY

THE HOSPITAL COMPLAINTS SYSTEM: WORKING IN WHOSE INTERESTS?

Women, on the whole, are not motivated by the desire for monetary compensation when they seek redress; they are much more likely to be seeking justice for themselves and their families and a restoration of their self-respect. They are very likely to have made a complaint through the Hospital Complaints System and found that route to be blocked by the medical profession and hospital administration – which always supports doctors against patients – before going to a solicitor. An unnecessary or unwanted hysterectomy is felt by some women to be such an intrusion, such an abuse, that they are likely to be 'driven' to find out why this was done. A woman who had been told she *had* to have a hysterectomy for a condition which turned out to be nothing to do with her womb, said to me, 'I would have been happy, with "I am sorry, we made a mistake", but they did everything they could to justify what they had done including changing what I had said in my hospital records, that in the end I was so angry and there was no way of redress left to me but to sue.'

Losing, falsifying, amending documents to suit the case of the doctor, citing the patient as an alcoholic and therefore an irresponsible patient, dubbing the patient hysterical and therefore mentally unstable and not to be believed as well as telling blatant lies about what has happened, are what women have to face when seeking redress either through the complaints system or through the civil courts. Everyone in the hospital, from the most lowly employee to the highest consultant, is sworn to protect the reputation of the doctors and this conspiracy of silence makes it difficult for the patient to obtain justice. No one in the hospital system dares speak out for the patient because if they do the medical mafia will ensure the end of their career.

GPs who should be advocates for the patient, often participate in this injustice, driving patients to the limits of their endurance. Delaying tactics are often used as well since a patient must bring a case of medical negligence against a doctor or hospital within a limit of three years. Under the Health Records Act 1990 patients are entitled to have access to their medical records, both the hospital's and their GP's, and these must be supplied within forty calendar days. The patient has to apply to the hospital and the surgery for them, paying a small fee for access and for the cost of photocopying the documents.

SEEKING REDRESS THROUGH SOLICITORS

Solicitors can obtain the records for the patient but they apply for them under a different Act of Parliament, The Administration of Justice Act 1970, but under this Act there is no time limit allocated for delivery of the documents. This allows hospital, doctors and advocates to 'sit' on the documents and spin out the time during which the patient has to bring the case. The patient's solicitor will have to go to the High Court to get a judicial ruling that the hospital must supply the records within a certain period of time before they can progress the case for the patient. This whole process may take many months of crucial time; indeed it has been known to take more than a year for a patient to get access to her NHS hospital and doctor's notes. By these means, doctors and hospitals prevent patients from enjoying two of the rights, numbers 3 and 6, embodied in the Patients Charter, the Bill of Rights for Patients:

3. To have any complaint about NHS services – whoever provides them – investigated and to receive a prompt written reply from the chief executive or general manager.
6. To have access to health records, and to know that those working for the NHS are under a legal duty to keep their contents confidential.

The documents are rarely supplied to the patient or the patient's solicitor unvetted; it is usual for the hospital and the GP records and documents to be carefully studied to minimize any incriminating evidence. The solicitors working for the hospital will vet the documents which are to be sent to the patient's solicitors, but when patients apply for the records themselves, it is likely to be a clerk, hospital administrator or surgery manager who carries out this task. Doctors sometimes vet the documents themselves, though this is generally regarded as unethical by the medical profession. Because solicitors apply for the documents under a High Court ruling, there is less likelihood that the vetting solicitors will be heavy-handed. Specialist medical litigation solicitors have become expert at being able to detect whether documents have been altered, replaced, added to or removed and evidence of this kind is often cited in court cases.

Under the Patients Charter, NHS patients have rights which are the focus of many negligence legal cases. Two of these, numbers 4 and 5, are rights which apply to informed consent and second referrals:

4. To be referred to an acceptable consultant, when the GP thinks it is necessary, and to be referred for a second opinion if patient and GP agree that is desirable.
5. To be given a clear explanation of any treatment proposed, including any risks and any alternatives before agreement to treatment.

SEEKING REDRESS

It is the flouting and denial of these two rights which leads to many cases of medical litigation. The law of consent states that an agreement must be one made with full understanding and information; in other words, there is no legal consent if, for whatever reason, pertinent information is withheld. Many doctors, however, feel that they have a superior duty to keep painful information away from the patient even if, by doing so, they are not complying with the law. A cancer specialist writing in the medical journal, *The Lancet*, said that 'doctors may sometimes be justified in telling white lies to patients to reassure them they are not suffering from a disease which they have always dreaded.'[1] Taken to its extremes, this belief in a calling above the law could allow a doctor to tell lies to the patient as a means of securing an operation which may be of financial benefit to the doctor. As one patient put it, 'What is the difference between God and a gynaecologist? God doesn't think he is a gynaecologist!'

The Royal College of Surgeons is alerting patients of their rights in relation to surgery by producing a booklet on the subject of informed consent called 'Consent to Surgery' which they intend to issue to patients. They are, wrongly in my opinion, placing the emphasis on the consentee to ensure that the law is properly applied. I feel that there will be no improvement in the application of the law of consent until it is rigorously applied by the medical profession and for that reason it would be more appropriate to direct a pamphlet to doctors who regularly infringe the consent law. There is no justification for doctors avoiding, deflecting, bending or ignoring the law of consent in relation to their patients. It is absolutely right that patients should be given accurate information – neither dressed up nor dressed down – about their condition as well as full information on treatments and their consequences. An agreement to work within the law of consent should be built into the conditions and terms of contract. Furthermore, I believe that abuse in gynaecology is so rife that *deliberately* not applying the law of

consent by gynaecologists, wherever this is detected, should be an
offence meriting instant dismissal.

CIVIL LAW AND MEDICAL NEGLIGENCE

There is no statute law which covers medical litigation so a
patient has to bring a case under civil law to sue the doctor and the
hospital for compensation. Bringing a case of medical negligence is
one of the most difficult types of cases to prove. It is also fraught with
problems simply because so much of the interaction between doctors
and patients goes unrecorded, therefore evidence usually settles on
what the doctor and the patient *perceived* to be said and *perceived* to be
the case, and on what the solicitor can detect through medical notes.
These cases require more than a perfect understanding of the law,
they require a great deal of specialist medical knowledge.
Gynaecological cases are significantly more difficult again because
the issues are often not as clear-cut as in other cases of medical
negligence, and many cases founder through lack of evidence
and the inexperience of solicitors.

Before a case of medical negligence can be brought the solicitor
has to find two expert witnesses – doctors working in the same
medical discipline – who will 'find for' the litigant. In other words, the
solicitor has to find two gynaecologists who will study the documents
and say that actions performed by the patient's gynaecologist were
unusual and not standard practice. It is the expert witness principle
in medical litigation, the Bolem precedent, which can also so easily
scupper a litigant's case. The hospital or doctor has only to find two
'responsible' gynaecologists who will testify that they would have
done the same thing in the same circumstances for the litigant's case
to be lost. Much depends on the solicitor being able to find additional
and incontrovertible evidence to support the litigant. When the
solicitor is satisfied that there is a 'good case' – one that has more

than a 50/50 chance of winning – they will take the case on and
formally issue a writ, a declaration to sue the doctor or hospital
for compensation.

FUNDING LEGAL ACTION

Funding legal action is also difficult. Basically there are
three methods: Legal Aid, self-funded, and 'No win no fee'.

Legal Aid is highly prized but extremely difficult to obtain.
A person who has a job with an income of more than £7,000 per
year and savings of more than £3,000 – unless he or she has a large
mortgage, a number of dependants and heavy family expenses – is
unlikely to get Legal Aid. The Legal Aid Board lays down guidelines as
to how much a person needs to live on, and what is left is 'disposable
income'. Disposable income and capital are used to assess
entitlement to Legal Aid. If Legal Aid is awarded by the Board, any
capital above £3,000 will be required as a down payment to the Board,
and a monthly sum, dependent on the litigant's disposable income,
will be required to be paid to the Board. Legal Aid is not free and the
cost of legal action over and above what is paid to the Board by the
litigant, will be recouped from the amount the litigant wins at the
end of the day.

Legal Aid protects the litigant against having to pay the other
side's costs if the case is lost and this is its main benefit. All the legal
costs, including the solicitor's fees, are paid for by the Legal Aid Board
with the exception of some restrictions on the type of costs which
can be incurred.

The cost of bringing a simple action for compensation which is
settled out of court will be in the region of £10,000, but this cost could
escalate to as much as £100,000 if the case goes to court. One woman
found that her household insurance through the Legal Protection
Group provided her with £25,000 of cover which was enough to bring

her case. Some medical litigation solicitors will take cases on a 'no win no fee' basis – this means that they take a higher fee, but the costs are not recovered unless and until the case is won. The litigant has to take out an insurance policy to insure against loss.

COMPLAINTS' PROCEDURES

There are three other actions which allow patient redress: making a complaint through the NHS complaints procedure; making a complaint to the Health Service Ombudsman; and making a complaint to the General Medical Council.

Issuing a complaint about treatment within the NHS is as difficult and as tortuous as suing and involves the patient in endless communication – letters, reports, statements. The Patients Charter states that any complaint must be investigated and a full and prompt written reply supplied by the chief executive or general manager. The problem lies in the interpretation of the words 'full' and 'investigation'. I know from my own experience, and from others who have been at the receiving end of these communications, that the explanation provided by the chief executive is nothing more than a word-for-word repetition of the doctor's own account and there is no attempt at an independent investigation. The report from the hospital is likely to be as far from a 'full investigation' as you can get. I found all of the letters I received from the chief executive very distressing because they just seemed to whitewash the hospital and put me in the wrong. Patients can enlist the help of the Community Health Council (CHC) in communicating with the hospital. Community Health Councils are independent bodies established in every health authority to act for and deal with patients' complaints. The CHC can complain on the behalf of the patient as well as arrange for the chief executive and the gynaecologist to meet the patient face to face to answer questions. Patients can insist on a fuller report if what is supplied is not satisfactory, and the hospital is obliged to produce one. The chief executive of the hospital is able to refer the case to the Consultant in Charge of Clinical Complaints at the Regional Health Authority for an Independent Professional Review. Patients who have taken this route rarely find that the report sheds any new light on their case. The Health Services Ombudsman is the ultimate complaints' body within the NHS for complaints about failures in administration when all the other avenues have failed.

The General Medical Council (GMC) is the doctors' disciplinary body, consisting of both doctors and lay people. It assesses the complaints of patients and, if necessary, takes action against the doctor. The ultimate discipline is for a doctor to be barred from practising medicine – struck off the medical register. Patients who bring actions have to send sworn statements to the GMC. Complaints are heard by the disciplinary panel and evidence is presented in open sessions very similar to a court hearing. Women have been heartened in recent years by the much more responsive approach by the GMC to their complaints against doctors.

9

Good advice and alternative health remedies

All the advice in the world will not be of any benefit to women unless they start off with the belief that it is *they*, and *they* alone, who have the right to decide what happens to *their* bodies. Whenever a woman sees any kind of therapist or doctor they *must* remember this important fact. When I saw my gynaecologist, the small voice inside me – call it whatever you want, intuition, common sense – said NO, NO, DON'T DO IT and I told the doctors in no uncertain terms that I would not have the castrating operation they had lined up for me. But I crumbled in the face of pressure and persuasion and I allowed them to bully me into having the operation *they wanted to give me*, not the treatment I wanted to have.

STRATEGIES FOR EMPOWERMENT

Women can only adopt a strong and determined attitude if they empower themselves, and that means acquiring knowledge. Reading this book is the first step towards achieving this empowerment. Gynaecologists are used to women deferring to them and they enjoy the power they are able to exert over them. Good gynaecologists are aware of this power, but do not abuse it, but the worst are men who are just 'hooked on power'. The best antidote is to diffuse their power with a few strategems and positive thinking, so you can make the interaction between the gynaecologist and yourself one between equals. The following 20 strategies will help you achieve this.

1. First and foremost NEVER go to see anyone about your gynaecological problems on your own. Always take your partner, or a friend, sister, mother, etc. The person who accompanies you is there to be your support and your witness as to what is said in the consultation. Whoever accompanies you must be with you throughout the whole of the consultation, including the examination. GPs are used to patients taking someone to the surgery, but consultants invariably invent their own rules about what they will and will not allow.

    A friend of mine, a very strong and self-assured young woman who has severe endometriosis, has had many consultations with gynaecologists and she always takes her husband with her. She has attended several hospitals and has seen several different specialists but has only once had an adverse reaction. The gynaecologist at her local hospital obviously did not like her husband being present, possibly because it restricted his opportunity to influence her, so he conducted the whole consultation in a completely bizarre way, speaking to her through her husband and not addressing her at all. At the end of the consultation he very kindly offered her a hysterectomy which she immediately refused.

2. **Do not see any doctor who refuses to allow you to have your witness with you.** It is a perfectly reasonable request, and a sensible thing to do as it will make you feel much more comfortable about the consultation. The right to have someone with you is worth fighting for, so if it is refused make a point of complaining to your Community Health Council about the doctor. If the doctor says that he/she will conduct only part of the consultation with the witness in the room, tell him or her politely that you wish your witness to be present for moral support for the whole of the consultation and that you will not continue the consultation without them present. Only leave after making every effort to persuade the consultant to agree. Make an appointment to see your GP immediately and tell him/her what has happened. Make sure that the GP understands that you will only see a consultant who allows you to have your witness present. Your GP should then refer you to another consultant.

3. **Always make sure that you have thought about the consultation in advance.** You should have some firm ideas about what you are prepared to let the gynaecologist do to you and what you will definitely not agree to. If you have any questions you want to ask, make sure that you write them down and take them with you. The consultant will have much more respect for you if he/she can see that you have made some effort to prepare yourself for the meeting. Make sure that you and your witness take notebooks with you and that you both write down the answers to your questions. This is important because it is well known that patients do not take in all that is being said to them in consultations, particularly if what the doctor is saying is distressing. 'YOU HAVE GOT TO HAVE A HYSTERECTOMY' definitely falls into this category. Writing down the answers will also focus your mind. Adopting an attitude of detachment is a very good thing to do anyway; just imagine that it is someone else the doctor is talking about and not you, and this will enable you to think more rationally about what is being said and enable you to ask purposeful questions. One patient I know is so wary of doctors that she always takes a tape recorder with her when she goes to see a consultant,

and she tells me that only one doctor has refused to allow her to use it. A tape recording would be very useful if, for example, clarification was needed about what was or was not said in the consultation.

4. **If, for example, you have decided in advance to say no to a hysterectomy,** say this to your GP or consultant at the outset of the meeting, so they are in no doubt about your views. The discussion should then centre around what could be offered that will be acceptable to you. If you are offered an endometrial ablation or myomectomy, you will want to find out how experienced the gynaecologist is in doing them because these are tricky operations. Tell him/her that you know that patients have died having endoscopic and laparoscopic surgery, so you want to know how many he/she has done in the past. Make sure that you get a proper answer to the question. The gynaecologist will not be happy about you taking this line of enquiry, but it is your right to know. If you meet anger or hostility, just ask him/her, 'Would you like to be driven on a motorway by someone who did not have a driving licence?'

5. **Be ready with all your arguments** as the consultant will probably try to persuade you to accept a hysterectomy, simply because that is all that most of them can do. The gynaecologist will almost certainly talk to you about the risks of developing womb or ovarian cancer and will try to convince you that you ought to take advantage of having a hysterectomy to prevent it. However if this is not what you want just tell him or her politely that you will expect to be given evidence that you have got cancer and by that you mean copies of all the reports and tests carried out.

6. **Do not take an expression like 'we cannot rule out cancer ...', or 'there is a risk of ...'** to mean that you actually do have cancer. Be warned, these expressions mean nothing at all. Far too often gynaecologists say that cancer 'may be present' when there is none at all. There is only one question to as, 'Do I have cancer or not?' Make sure you get a straight answer to that

question and of course tell them that you will expect to be given proof. As I have already shown, the chances of you actually having cancer are quite small, but it does remain a possibility. If you are told you definitely have cancer keep a cool head and demand proof as there is still a possibility they have got it wrong, or they are planning a prophylactic operation. Under the Health Records Act 1990 you are entitled to see your medical records; use this right and demand to see biopsy reports and every test and examination that is carried out on you. It is your body and you have the right to be properly informed about what is wrong with you.

If a positive test is discovered as a result of a cervical smear, you will be wise to find out the cause and what treatment may be needed, as these tests are carried out independently. Modern conservative laser treatment for abnormal cells does not mean surgery. If there is pronounced cancer, surgery on the cervix does not need to be a major operation such as a hysterectomy. A cone biopsy (localised operation) on the cervical canal will be enough to remove the cancerous tissues if the cancer is not pronounced and widespread. Always make sure that you are offered the conservative option. There are still gynaecologists who will want to do a hysterectomy for cervical cancer and this is totally unwarranted.

7. **You have the right to decide!** Remember that doctors are professional people, just like lawyers and accountants, employed to give advice that you are under no obligation to accept. They have no power to coerce, frighten, threaten or bully you into doing what you do not want. Doctors, and especially gynaecologists, assume a powerful attitude, as if they had some given right built into their terms and conditions of employment, to ensure that you have to have the treatment they specify. They do not have such a right. You alone have the right to accept or refuse any treatment offered. Your GP has no right at all to threaten to strike you off his/her list if you will not take this advice. If you should refuse treatment and your GP does threaten you with this action, then you must make a complaint to the Family Health Authority and Community Health Council. If you feel your

gynaecologist is pressurizing you into a hysterectomy, then you should make a complaint immediately to your Community Health Council.

8. **All women would benefit by becoming more assertive in dealing with doctors** rather than blanketly agreeing to the treatments they prescribe. The penalty for not asking questions can be, as I have shown in the case studies, death, or years of pain far more serious than that which led the patient to the doctor in the first place. I know I was not nearly assertive enough myself. I was swept along with a tide of emotion because I did not suspend my disbelief long enough. I was seduced by the aura of the 'respected medical profession'. This is a myth. A doctor is only as good as a doctor is. Some are very good and of benefit to their patients, and some are so bad that you would not wish them on your worst enemy.

   If I could have a wish it would be that my bad experience could be turned into something of value for other women, especially those who have not yet been touched by the gynaecological profession. Question doctors: it does not matter if they label you a 'difficult patient' and write this on your records. It is much better to have a label than to wind up unhappy and full of regrets.

9. **It is very important that your witness is with you particularly during the internal examination.** A nurse is supposed to be present, but you do still encounter hospitals where a male gynaecologist carries out this very personal examination without one there. You should never agree to this. Women have been known to be sexually abused by their doctors under the guise of an internal examination. Make sure that the examination is carried out in a way that is acceptable to you. I was subjected to an examination by a male gynaecologist when there was no nurse present which I found very degrading and humiliating and I complained about this to the hospital authorities.

10. **It is very important that the consultation is not hurried.** If the gynaecologist has only a few minutes, tell him that is not time enough. You deserve a longer consultation than that. Make an appointment to come back again and tell him/her that you expect to have at least forty-five minutes to discuss your condition. Make it clear that if the gynaecologist cannot spare adequate time, then you are not prepared to take the matter further. Please remember that your body is important to him/her too. Without it, they would be out of a job!

11. **You do not need to make a decision about treatment at the first consultation.** Tell the consultant that you want to go away and think about what has been said to you and that you may want to come back for a further consultation. There are very few conditions which require urgent treatment so give yourself plenty of time to think. Even if you are told you have cancer and urgent treatment is necessary, you should not suspend caution – make sure that they have not made a mistake in diagnosis or got the wrong patient notes. A lot of stupid mistakes could be prevented simply by the patient being more assertive with the doctor.

12. **After the consultation you and your witness should exchange notes** and together write an account which you both agree describes exactly what took place. This document will be very important to you when you next go to see the consultant and treatment possibilities are discussed with you more fully. It will also be pertinent if you agree to treatment and something goes wrong whilst you are being operated on or in the hospital.

13. **Get a second opinion** if you are not happy with what the gynaecologist suggests to you for whatever reason. You will have to go back to your GP to get this; under the Patients' Charter the GP will refer you for a second opinion only if you and he/she agree that this is desirable. Good GPs will be very happy to arrange a second opinion. But if your GP is reluctant to send you to another hospital, tell him or her that you will not have any treatment at all without having had a second opinion.

ADVICE AND ALTERNATIVES

✳ 14. **Members of the Campaign Against Hysterectomy and Unnecessary Operations on Women** are offered the opportunity of getting a second opinion from one of these experts. If you join the Campaign, which costs only a few pounds, you may well have access to a much better second opinion than your GP will offer you and you may find, as many women have, that you do not need an operation at all.

15. **A good gynaecologist will do a pregnancy test as routine** before carrying out an internal examination or performing surgery, but there have been many tragic cases where women have lost their babies because this simple precaution has not been carried out. If you are at any risk, however slight, of being pregnant, do a test yourself.

✳ 16. **Once you are convinced that surgery, either major or minor, is essential, make sure you know exactly what is being proposed.** For example, are they intending to do an investigation, a laparoscopy or hysteroscopy, or perform surgery? Amazingly, gynaecologists are extremely vague about this. Gynaecologists like to be given complete carte blânche to do whatever they want. Do not give them this right. You must be absolutely clear about what it is they are planning to do. Your full and informed consent should be sought, but this is often 'fudged' and the proposed actions of the gynaecologist not made clear.

✳ 17. **Make sure that the gynaecologist tells you about all the risks and possible complications** of the operation, and what he/she will do to reduce them. Ask him/her about their previous operative complications and how he/she has dealt with them and also to put a risk factor on your particular surgical procedure. If the gynaecologist begins to get irritable at this line of enquiry, ask if he or she would have surgery without knowing the consequences. I have no doubt that questioning of this sort will put the doctor 'on guard' and make him or her more careful in the operating theatre.

THE CASE AGAINST HYSTERECTOMY

18. **Make sure that you see and read the patients' consent form** which gives
your consent to surgery, so that when you sign it you are absolutely aware
of what you are agreeing to. All too often the consent form, delivered by a
junior doctor when the patient has already been admitted to the hospital
and is therefore very vulnerable, is not given to the patient to read, but only
to sign. This is, in my opinion, an abuse in itself. The form should be sent
together with the hospital admission papers to your home so that you can
read and digest them. If there is anything in the consent form you do not like,
or would not consider in the course of surgery, then you must add this to it
in the form of a note written on the document at the appropriate place.

19. **The Campaign Against Hysterectomy** has produced its own consent to
surgery form (see Campaigning for better treatment, p. 104) which you can use
as well to back up your consent to surgery. This form declares unambiguously
what surgery you are agreeing to and what you are not. The form is intended
to be copied to the gynaecologist and hospital administrator and, if need be, to
the patient's solicitor. The Campaign Against Hysterectomy consent form will
provide vital evidence should anything go wrong during surgery.

20. **If you do have second thoughts about having surgery,** or you feel that not
enough information has been given to you, or you are unhappy about it, or
you just decide at a late stage against it, then you do not have to have it.
Simply tell them you do not want it. You can do this even if you have been
admitted to hospital. You can withdraw your consent right up to the last
minute before being given the anaesthetic. You may be embarrassed about
doing this, but believe me, it is much better to be embarrassed than to go
through with an operation you do not want and suffer the consequences.
You know now that the likelihood of anything serious happening to you if
you say no is quite small. Yes ... you might get cancer if you do not have a
hysterectomy, but you also might have an accident driving your car at night,
and the risk of that happening is much greater. However, we do not stop
driving our cars and nor should we have unnecessary hysterectomies.

ADVICE AND ALTERNATIVES

It should be possible for all healthy women who are suffering from nothing more than heavy periods or fibroids to go through life without ever seeing a gynaecologist, as women did in the past, before there was so much emphasis on abdominal surgery. Before doctors and hospital medicine became generally available, women would seek help from a variety of sources for the problems they experienced. Without taking a retrogressive step, women today should consider looking at these alternatives together with modern conservative and reconstructive surgery to find a solution which gives them the best of both worlds. For an increasing number of women, a mixture of herbalism or homeopathic medicine, improved diet and exercise, provides a solution to their problems. Support can also come from yoga and meditation, aromatherapy, autogenics (a relaxation technique), T'ai chi and acupuncture as all these are stress relievers and stress is known to be a trigger for painful periods. A diet which is low in fat, high in fibre and includes plenty of fresh fruit and vegetables, coupled with regular exercise, especially exercise centred on the pelvic area, is also seen to be very important in controlling these conditions. Fibroids grow more vigorously when the diet contains animal fats, cheese, eggs and fried foods. Alternative medicine can also provide effective treatments for endometriosis, ovarian cysts and cancer.

There is no doubt that many women find alternative medicine very helpful and they feel deeply reassured when a health prescription means they do not need to have major surgery. The very best treatment solution would be for specialists in alternative medicine to work together with gynaecologists using conservative surgical techniques. There is no doubt that such treatment would work for the benefit of *all* women and a united front such as this would both *prevent* and *cure* these conditions.

10

What you can do to help yourself

Generally speaking, good health has been proved to be directly related to the effort you make to keep well. Begin with the idea that you *can* affect your wellbeing – and that includes all parts of your body, including your womb and your ovaries. Oddly enough, women have the notion that these parts are not affected by general health programmes, so nothing can be done to prevent or help fibroids, painful and heavy menstrual bleeding, or even cancer, except to opt for surgery. This is not true. I do not want to give the impression that self-help remedies will completely do away with gynaecologists; this is clearly not the case if a problem is persistent, but I do think that if women were to try alternative remedies, then many, if not most, would end up not having to go to a doctor in the first place.

ATTENDING TO YOUR DIET

Begin by looking at your diet – is it good enough for you? By that I mean, does it contain a variety of foods with different nutritional values, vitamins and minerals? Is it low in fat, low in sugar, and high in fibre, with plenty of fresh fruits and vegetables? Then look at a programme of exercise; follow this up with stress-relieving strategies and lifestyle changes. And do all this long before you go to see your doctor so you give things a chance to work.

Many women contact me and tell me about their extreme menstrual pain and heavy periods, so I know how debilitating this can be and why some may feel that having a hysterectomy is the best thing for them – simply because it gets rid of the problem. I am a vegetarian and, for years before I was diagnosed as having an ovarian cyst which led to my operation, I was so dedicated to my job that I did not eat properly a lot of the time – a cheese and tomato sandwich, an apple and a cup of coffee for lunch and then back to work. When I got home at night I was too exhausted to cook a proper meal so I would make myself a snack which might well contain more cheese. I realize now that this diet was profoundly unbalanced and grossly lacking in some of the basic nutrients that I needed to make my body function properly. Although it was high in calcium, amino acids, Vitamins B_1, B_2, B_3, A and D, it was lacking in essential minerals like zinc, iron and magnesium, and Vitamins B_6, E and K_1 B_1, B_2, B_3, A and D are all vitamins which can be purchased separately or as complex pills in a health shop or chemist.[1] It was very heavily weighted towards animal fats which are known to be cystic. I took multi-vitamin supplements, Vitamin C, and B_{12} but this was not enough to replace the missing vitamins and minerals necessary to establish a hormonal balance. In actual fact, I was probably quite undernourished, and I felt tired and worn out. The iron in my multi-vitamin tablets was not enough to restore my haemoglobin to a normal level. (In anaemia the red cells are fewer, or have less haemoglobin than normal; haemoglobin is the pigment that gives red blood cells their colour). Anaemia leads to heavy bleeding. Taking iron pills and altering your diet to include more iron will help.

Looking after your health means making a commitment to changing those things in your life which tend to, or will, lead to future problems.[2] Essential fatty acids (EFAs) are part of a healthy diet; they fall into two groups – series 6, essential fatty acids, are extracted from sunflowers, corn, evening primrose, almonds, green vegetables and wholegrain cereals; and series 3, from fish, walnuts, rapeseed and soya beans. EFAs help with the absorption of calcium so they are important in the protection of bones. If you make a point of building regularly into your diet iron, calcium and magnesium supplements, in combination with vitamins A, C, B complex, D and E and B-carotene, contained in oranges, carrots and apricots, you will be protecting yourself against many of the problems caused by hormonal imbalance that may lead to a prescription for hysterectomy. Calcium and iron are particularly important as women get older and enter the peri-menopausal and menopause phases.

Government health warnings about diet concentrate on the issue of large amounts of animal fat because of the connection with heart disease and strokes. Is it reasonable then to suppose that these saturated fats can affect other parts of the body as well? Professor Campbell, an eminent gynaecologist, suggests in his book on fibroids that eating a healthy diet containing essential minerals like iron and magnesium, and essential fatty acids from vegetable oils, taken together with exercise to reduce body weight and oestrogen levels, helps in the reduction of heavy bleeding caused by fibroids.[3] No proper research has been done on the connection between diet and the health of the womb and ovaries; indeed it would be difficult to do. But such a study would be interesting and point to a cure for menorrhagia (heavy periods), dysmenorrhoea (painful periods) and possibly dyspareunia (painful intercourse) too. Meanwhile, we can only refer to the experiences of many women that an improved diet does reduce heavy menstrual bleeding. And research is currently being carried out to produce a medical therapy for menorrhagia.

HERBAL AND HOMEOPATHIC REMEDIES WIDELY AVAILABLE

There are a number of widely available patent and homeopathic remedies which some women find helpful. I would personally like to recommend evening primrose oil; many women have benefitted from this oil which is rich in series 6 essential fatty acids. I have been taking this for many months and have found my skin and hair improved and I feel altogether much calmer – hormonally balanced. I have also been taking a mixed mineral supplement of calcium, zinc and magnesium which has helped me mentally – I feel more alert and my memory is better. Zinc does have an effect on brain functioning and is used in the treatment of Alzheimer's disease. Ellen Grant says that, 'Zinc is crucial for the growth and division of cells, for brain development and function and indeed for the normal functioning of every single cell'.[4]

Medicinal herbalists and homeopathic doctors have been found to be very good too in dealing with all of the problems of the womb and ovaries and the ovulatory cycle. The end result of all these treatments, whether they are through traditional, alternative or complementary medicine, is to establish control over the conditions which cause pain and balance the system.

A herbalist will want to go into great detail with you about your menstrual cycle in order to find an exact treatment, so it is advisable to keep records. For example: you should keep a daily log and note down how you feel – when you feel good, when you feel depressed, the days when you have PMT and how that affects you, and the occurrence and type of menstrual pain, how long it lasts, whether it is a cramping type of short duration or a continuous aching pain, what you use to treat it, how this works and if there are side effects, such as nausea, etc., how long your period lasts, the onset day and the last day of bleeding, and exactly how you feel on those days.

You will find out from keeping detailed records whether your periods fall into a predictable pattern or whether they are variable and at what point in the cycle pain regularly occurs. Such information would also be invaluable to a good gynaecologist in pinpointing your problem. The time of menstrual pain in the cycle is a significant indicator as to whether the cause is endometriosis, hyperfolliculinemia (excessive oestrogen), and higher than normal concentrations of prostaglandin, a substance which promotes the contraction of the womb and menstrual pain. Pain which reaches its peak at the time of maximum flow is due to endometriosis. Adenomyosis will also result in excessive menstrual pain on the right side of the womb.[5]

I think that it would be a good thing if *every* woman with hormonal problems were to keep such a record. The more you know about your body and about your condition, about the treatments that are available and how to use the medical services, the better the outcome will be for you in terms of treatment.

THE IMPORTANCE OF REGULAR EXERCISE

Taking regular exercise is something else you can do to improve your general health, the health of your womb and ovaries, and your feeling of wellbeing. Exercise burns up calories and increases the metabolic rate, so the body functions more efficiently. It has also been shown to decrease menstrual pain, possibly due to the suppression of prostaglandins or by increasing the supply of endorphins to the body (endorphins are the body's painkillers).[6] Women who are overweight tend to produce too much oestrogen which causes heavy periods, large blood clots and extensive shedding of the lining of the womb.

Exercises to strengthen the abdominal wall are particularly valuable to women with an early indication of prolapse; by strengthening these muscles, a hysterectomy could be avoided.[7]

Dieting to lose weight is now frowned upon due to its effects on the body. At its most extreme, the consequences of anorexia nervosa and bulimia can be destructive of the body's hormonal and skeletal system. Dieting – as well as excessive exercise – can result in the whole ovulatory system shutting down. Both create a protein and fat deficiency which are harmful. The absence of oestrogen, normally released in menstruation, almost certainly affects the long-term health of the bones: the many women athletes who have developed osteoporosis are witness to this.[8] Nowadays dieting has given way to aerobic exercise as the best way to lose weight; and brisk walking, working out in a gym, running and cycling are all excellent forms of aerobic exercise, as well as very enjoyable activities in themselves.

Women's lives are extraordinarily full with too many conflicting roles leading to a high degree of stress. There is evidence to show that stress is a factor in the formation of ovarian cysts and that it contributes to menstrual pain by stimulating the adrenal glands, thus causing an increase in cortisol and the amount of prostaglandin produced.[9] Reflexology, aromatherapy and acupuncture can be of great benefit in dealing with pain and physical stress and stress-relieving exercise programmes, such as yoga and T'ai chi, bring about inner composure. Vitamin B_6 also helps to restore balance.[10] Women suffering from depression, for example, have been found to be deficient in Vitamin B_6. Autogenic (mind control) exercises and games and puzzles, which induce a measure of mental control, are stress-relieving too![11]

If you have been diagnosed as suffering from endometriosis or osteoporosis, joining the appropriate specialist society will be very helpful to you. They are expert in the understanding and treatment of sufferers, and have access to specialists who will be able to assess you independently from your local hospital. You will also be guaranteed the very latest treatment advice. It will certainly be worth the few pounds to join. (Details of these and other organizations are given under 'Where to Go for Advice and Help', p. 111.) There is a new treatment for endometriosis which can remove the endometrial tissue in the pelvic area with laparoscopic surgery using laser fibre technology, but it is only available at a few hospitals.

THINK TWICE ABOUT DRUGS

What is known about the use of hormone-containing drugs – the Pill, HRT and fertility drugs – is that they interfere with the take-up of minerals and nutrients, and there is a definite connection between these drugs and cancer.[12] Whilst I would not dispute the value of HRT to women who have had their ovaries removed to help, or prevent them from developing osteoporosis, they should be aware that there is a risk involved. My personal feeling is that it is wise to keep away from them if you can. There are naturally occurring oestrogens – available from soya beans and soya products, alfalfa, ginseng, celery, fennel and other green and yellow vegetables, as well as from red clover, rhubarb, linseeds, liquorice, anise and the herb, dong quai – which will provide enough oestrogens for most menopausal women without resorting to drugs.[13]

Taking cortisone drugs over a long period causes depletion of bone density, as does excessive dieting, over-exercising, smoking heavily and drinking alcohol and caffeine to excess.[14] If you fall into any of these categories, you will be wise to ask your GP for a bone-density scan. Oophorectomized post-menopausal women are most at risk and they should insist that such a scan is made available to them. Women with osteoporosis do have to be particularly vigilant of their health because of the danger of a fracture or broken bone. Impact exercise, such as walking or running, is absolutely essential to keep bones healthy, as well as taking calcium and vitamin supplements regularly.

WHAT YOU CAN DO TO HELP YOURSELF

Hysterectomy abroad
and women's rights

The *Sunday Times* revealed in a scoop story in 1994 that
three out of four operations carried out in the United Kingdom were
unnecessary. The study, which showed amongst other things, huge
regional variations in the number of hysterectomies performed said
that 'they could not be put down to anything but the different beliefs
of surgeons and preventative rituals which have no particular result'.
The surgeons' professional body, The Royal College of Surgeons,
caught off-guard by this exposure, quickly responded by saying,
'There is a great problem of medical uncertainty – there is an
urgent need for research.'

The 'problem of medical uncertainty', is that it centres around
the 'clinical judgement' of doctors and is not governed by any
overriding theories about treatment. 'Clinical judgement' varies from
doctor to doctor and from country to country.[1] In fact, what a doctor
or a surgeon does is much more related to where he grew up and
what his own personal views are than to any scientific evaluation

of symptoms or thoroughgoing concern for diagnosis. There is no national or international consensus about hysterectomy, nor about other areas of medicine, simply because beliefs about surgical procedures depend, not on symptoms or operative benefits, but on cultural attitudes in medicine and in society at large. For this reason, the French, who are much more concerned about the whole constitution of the patient, perform few hysterectomies, and the Americans, who are more interested in symptoms and diagnosis, perform a great many.

HYSTERECTOMY IN THE USA

Hysterectomy has never been an obsession in Europe as it has been in the United States. At the height of the hysterectomy craze, it was estimated that one in two women over the age of 40 had lost her womb.[2] By the late seventies and early eighties, women had started to question this medical ethos and a groundswell of resistance formed around HERS – the Hysterectomy Education and Research Society. HERS lobbied for legislation on consent and made women better informed about the causes and conditions which led to a prescription for hysterectomy. HERS produced literature and information on the operation and its consequences as well as setting up a clinic to provide a referral centre for patients who had been prescribed a hysterectomy. The result has been that many American women are rejecting hysterectomy and it is now in steep decline after a period of exceptional growth.

AND IN CANADA

Canada also had a high hysterectomy rate. It trailed the USA in the 1970s, but spiralled in the 1980s.[3] Concern about rising public health costs by the Saskatchewan Department of Health and Welfare

checked the rise with a new approach: every recommendation
for hysterectomy was referred to an expert panel from the College
of Physicians and Surgeons who adjudicated as to whether the
operation was justified or not. The second line referral system, which
has been the main advantage of the French system, has proved to be
a very effective means of reducing the hysterectomy rate in Canada –
in fact, it dropped by one third in four years. The main benefit of a
system like this is that it has the potential to iron out differences
between regions and hospitals and doctors. Regional hysterectomy
rates in the United Kingdom vary by as much as four times from
region to region, and between hospital to hospital from 5 per cent to
40 per cent.[4] Where the regional rate is low, there is a danger that
women who need treatment may not be able to get it, and where it is
too high, women will be having unnecessary operations and public
money will be wasted.

THE UK'S INCREASING RATE

The reduction in the number of hysterectomies in Canada and
the United States is in sharp contrast to the United Kingdom where
the number has increased by 25 per cent over the last 15 years until it
is now the most performed operation on women, after abortion, both
in the NHS and in private practice.[5] In fact, the United Kingdom is the
only country in the world which has an *increasing* hysterectomy rate.
Even so, the UK with a rate of about 30 per cent is still not as high as
the United States, (50 per cent), but if current trends persist then it is
possible that the UK will overtake the US before too long.[6] Compared
to every other European country, the UK stands alone for this large
scale mutilation of women. Of the 29 million women and girls in the
United Kingdom, one in five will have lost her womb by the time she
reaches 65 at the current rate of operation: at present, 28 women out
of every 10,000 have a hysterectomy. In Norway only eleven out of

10,000 women have lost their womb, whereas Sweden has a rate of thirteen out of 10,000. German women are more usually treated with a wide range of drugs taken from both homeopathic, herbal and medical drugs registers, and if a hysterectomy is performed it is much more likely to be a vaginal operation.

THE FRENCH MODEL

A much more civilised regime prevails in France where no woman under forty would be given a hysterectomy for fibroids, for example, as gynaecologists would always choose to perform a myomectomy. The French model is undoubtedly the best in the world and results in only a fraction of the number of hysterectomies being performed compared to the United States, and of all gynaecological operations 70 per cent are conservative surgery.[7] And the hysterectomy itself is much more likely to be a sub-total operation, leaving the cervix in place. The French, with their holistic approach to medicine, view the deciding factor for removing a womb as being the presence of a life-threatening disease. French doctors are more likely than other doctors in Europe to be trained in conventional as well as homeopathic medicine and they are just as likely to prescribe vitamins and herbal therapies to patients.[8] The separation of gynaecology from obstetrics and medicinal treatments from surgery in gynaecology has meant that there are more filtering points for treatment which has worked for the benefit of French women. However, due to the recession, the public health system in France is now under threat.

From the 1960s the rapid growth in the number of consultant gynaecologist appointments in the United Kingdom meant that by the early 1980s the increase rate stood at one and a half times.[9] The national birth rate dropped by one third during this period – with the result that a decline in obstetric work left gynaecologists looking for other avenues for their skills. It should come as no surprise, then, that the rapid increase in the hysterectomy rate coincides almost exactly with this period.[10] British patients tend to be more ignorant about their bodies than, for example, the average French patient. Because of this, UK doctors diagnose and treat more, and yet do far fewer screening tests.[11] Diagnosis is therefore more likely to be a hit and miss affair compared to, say, the United States. UK doctors are also very resistant to change, to taking up new ideas, new types of treatment or new operative procedures, even if of benefit to their patients.[12] Furthermore, compared to other countries, caring by doctors in the United Kingdom is paternalistic and British patients have far fewer rights than their counterparts in France, Germany or the USA.[13] In a survey, one-third of patients said they would never consider questioning their doctors, and one-fifth were afraid to do so in case of a hostile reaction.[14] The right to see our medical records, a right which American patients have had for many years, has been available in the UK only in the last five years. Such curbs on personal liberty would not be tolerated in the United States where women have secured far greater freedom than anywhere else in the world.[15] It is more than curious, then, that it is these very same women who are so vulnerable to hysterectomy. The history of the women's movement has shown that acquiring the freedoms which have been won has not been easy. Freedom from unnecessary operations – surgical freedom – if it is to be achieved, will follow the same path as the achievements of other freedoms for women: namely that it will have to be fought for and won for women by women.

THE STRUGGLE FOR WOMEN'S RIGHTS

The first wave of women's liberation began in the mid-nineteenth century with the struggle for the vote. By the the early twentieth century the movement for women's suffrage had stepped up their actions. The First World War intervened but in 1918 Parliament gave the vote to all women over thirty.[16] In 1928 under the Women's Suffrage Reform Act, the vote was given to all women over twenty-one; women finally had equal voting rights with men.[17] In 1919 Parliament passed the Sex Disqualification Removal Act which allowed women to sit on juries and serve in local government.

Fifty years later, with the second wave of women's liberation and changes for women largely brought about through sexual liberation and the Pill, women began to feel that they were stakeholders in society but they still wanted to play a bigger part. In Britain, women's liberation effected a number of mould-breaking acts of Parliament – equal pay, sex discrimination, abortion, family law, child support – and paved the way for a tremendous growth in education and employment opportunities for women.

In spite of these changes, and even with the great increase in the number of women taking up medicine, behaviour of doctors towards patients has not altered. Women still have no rights over their own bodies – with the exception of abortion which is protected by law. It is curious that we have tolerated this for so long, and that we should continue to tolerate it at a time when women are more assertive and better educated than ever. A woman can run a company but she cannot decide what happens to her body on the operating table ... and doctors continue to make decisions for us just as if women's liberation had never happened.

It is almost impossible now to imagine how restrictive life was in the 1950s when a woman's role was absolutely defined by house and home, and very few women experienced higher education. Then the prevalent pattern for the treatment of gynaecological problems was closer to the French than to the American model. Women were more likely to have been given a 'tonic' for heavy menstrual bleeding and a myomectomy for fibroids. In the intervening years, the UK seems to have moved closer to the US model, with an aggressively increasing number of operations, less than 10 per cent of which are for malignancies, and one-half of which are performed on women under forty-five. That women have been timid in accepting these operations goes without saying. They have been willing to accept the judgement of doctors on the grounds that 'they are doctors and they should know'.

But the truth is now out, and women will no longer accept the operations gynaecologists choose to perform on us. Doctors will no more be able to tell us that it may be uncomfortable, but it will be *good for us* in the end. Giving a pain to effect a cure has always been the mainstay of an old-fashioned British male doctor attitude to life which is not acceptable to women today. Women all over the country have come to believe that what has been done to them has not been good; in fact, it has been brutal, and they are demanding a change. The third wave of the liberation of women will be now, and it will the liberation of women from surgical abuse.

PART 3

Summing up

12

Proof positive against hysterectomy

In summing up, I would like to reiterate nine questions about hysterectomy and the case against it.

- Are there too many hysterectomies?
- Is hysterectomy a good treatment?
- Are hysterectomies performed as a result of wrong diagnosis or prejudice?
- Are there too many gynaecologists?
- Are women being undermined by hysterectomy?
- Are too many hysterectomies performed on younger women?
- Do women have any rights over their bodies?
- Is public money being wasted?
- Can current practice be changed?

I trust that my evidence throughout this book has convinced you that there are far too many hysterectomies despite the efficacy of conservative surgical techniques and medical and alternative therapies. The negative effects of hysterectomy are far too great and the recovery time is far too long for it to be the mainstay of gynaecological treatment.

I trust the case studies and the comments of women themselves indicate strongly that hysterectomy has been a bad experience for many patients – that it is a risky procedure, and that for many, if the pros and cons and risk factors had been properly presented then no treatment at all would have been preferred. For the majority of women, the problems they suffer from are caused by hormonal imbalance and all of these conditions can be treated by medical, herbal, homeopathic and stress-relieving therapies.

I have submitted evidence that gynaecological diagnosis is very poor, that too few tests are carried out, and that mistakes in diagnosis are common, leading to a high number of unnecessary operations.

I do not believe that there are enough good gynaecologists and yet too many are employed for the work that ought to constitute good practice. There is some evidence to show that operations are prescribed purely to justify the existence of the gynaecologist and to provide a supplementary source of income from private work.

I believe that hysterectomy – the routine disregarding and underestimating of the effect that it, and especially oophorectomy, has on women – is an attack on the female psyche. The constant minimising of the effect of the operation has meant that there is no provision or help for the patient post-operatively, no counselling services available, no help for husbands, partners or families who have also to suffer the traumatic effects of hysterectomy and oophorectomy on women.

The evidence is overwhelming that hysterectomy is being performed on younger and younger women – more than half of the operations are on women under forty-five – that as a consequence these women are dependent over a long period of time on HRT for the protection of their bones, and yet this carries a known increased risk of breast cancer. There is also greater risk from heart attacks and strokes, an increased risk of premature ageing of the macula lutea of the eye and premature ageing of body, skin and bones. And hysterectomy can rob women of their chance to have children as more women delay doing so until they are in their thirties or forties.

As yet, there is no statute in law which defines and protects women from surgical abuse and the operations performed without informed consent are a denial of their human rights as women.

I have presented information about the exorbitant costs of current gynaecological practice: not only might 90 per cent of hysterectomies be unnecessary as well as 70 per cent of staff employed, but at a conservative estimate, £400 million of public money is wasted each year.

13

Gynaecologists and hospitals in the news

*Malcolm Pearce, Isaac Manyonda, Professor Geoffrey Chamberlain,
St George's Hospital, Tooting, London*

In 1994 two leading gynaecologists, Mr Malcolm Pearce and Professor Geoffrey Chamberlain, were involved in a fake pioneering operation at St George's Hospital, Tooting. Mr Pearce claimed in two papers submitted to *The Journal of Obstetrics and Gynaecology* that he had removed an ectopic pregnancy and implanted it through the cervix into the womb of a twenty-nine year old African woman, but this was entirely false. Professor Chamberlain, then the President of the Royal College of Obstetrics and Gynaecologists, who claimed he had given his name to the reports 'out of kindness', was forced to resign from the college. In 1995, Professor Chamberlain and Mr Isaac Manyonda, a Gynaecological Registrar at St George's, both listed as co-authors of the papers, were criticised for not checking the research by the chairman of the disciplinary committee of the General Medical Council, and Mr Pearce was struck off the medical register.

Sources: Daily Telegraph, British Medical Journal

All Saints Hospital, Chatham

In 1995 damages of £214, 206 were paid to the family of Susan Bielby, aged thirty-four, who died from cervical cancer in 1993. Her gynaecologist at All Saints Hospital, Chatham, described her pain due to an 'over-energetic sex life and self-abuse'. Her smear test in 1988 was positive and if this had been acted upon she could well have been cured.

Source: Daily Mail

Reginald Dixon, King's Mill Hospital, Sutton in Ashfield, Nottinghamshire

Reginald Dixon, Consultant Gynaecologist at King's Mill Hospital, Nottinghamshire, appeared before Mansfield magistrates charged with unlawfully procuring a miscarriage on Barbara Whiten. Mrs Whiten, aged thirty-five, believed she was infertile, so agreed to a hysterectomy. In the course of performing the operation Mr Dixon aborted her twelve-week foetus. The case was taken up by the Crown Prosecution Service. In 1995 Mr Dixon was tried under the 1967 Abortion Act at the Crown Court in Nottingham and was found not guilty. Mr Dixon admitted in Court that the abortion was a mistake.

King's Mill Hospital, Sutton in Ashfield, Nottinghamshire

Amanda Flewitt, twenty-nine, also found that she had been pregnant when she attended the King's Mill Hospital. She lost the baby when she had a gynaecological examination and discovered she had miscarried only when she was asked to return to the hospital for a scan.

Jane Henson, forty, also lost a baby at the King's Mill Hospital. She discovered after she had a hysterectomy that she had been pregnant.

Sources: Independent, Daily Telegraph, Daily Mail, Guardian

John Studd, Chelsea and Westminster Hospital, London

Leading Harley Street Gynaecologist, John Studd, a Consultant Gynaecologist at the Chelsea and Westminster Hospital, was sued by thirty-five year old Jaqui Bartley for removing her ovaries without consent in a private operation. She discovered their removal only when she received the bill for hormone replacement therapy. In 1995 Mrs Bartley won £32,500 damages and costs after the High Court ruled that Studd had acted unlawfully.

Sources: *Daily Telegraph, Guardian*

Walsgrave Hospital Trust, Coventry

In 1995 Sandra Masters was admitted to hospital as a day patient for laser treatment to her womb. During the operation the laser cut through her womb and colon, but she was discharged from hospital. She was readmitted with blood poisoning but her condition deteriorated and she suffered a major heart attack, leading to severe brain damage. The hospital has admitted liability.

Source: *Daily Telegraph*

Michael Pugh, Princess Grace Hospital, London

In 1995 Carole Burwash, fifty-three, was recommended to have a hysterectomy because for two years she had been suffering from severe menopausal symptoms. She was admitted to the private Princess Grace Hospital and the operation appeared to go well. After the operation, she was given an epidural injection to relieve her of pain but instead of a 3mg injection a mistake was made, and a 30mg dosage was given. She was rushed to the Middlesex Hospital but they could not save her.

Source: *Daily Telegraph*

Nicholas Siddle, University College Hospital, London

Nicholas Siddle was struck off the medical register in 1995 for damaging the organs of seven women, five during keyhole surgery. The GMC's medical conduct committee said that his care had fallen 'grossly below the standards patients were entitled to expect'. He was found to have performed keyhole surgery without adequate training in these techniques, leaving one women with a one-inch hole in her bladder and others with damaged urethras or perforated bowels.

Sources: Daily Telegraph

Nathaniel Adu, Luton and Dunstable Hospital

Nathaniel Adu was found guilty of serious professional misconduct and struck off the medical register in 1995, as a result of removing the healthy ovary of Mrs Vanessa King during a hysterectomy when she had written on the consent form 'left ovary not to be removed'.

Sources: Daily Telegraph, Daily Express

Raymond Garry, South Cleveland Hospital, South Tees Health Authority

Rita Walker, aged thirty-two, was awarded damages of £22,500 in 1995, after she was left with a damaged kidney as a result of 'pioneering' keyhole surgery, and her ovaries were removed unnecessarily. The health authority admitted liability.

Source: Daily Mail

Peter Dougherty, New Hall Hospital, Salisbury

Frances Henton, aged forty-seven, successfully sued gynaecologist Peter Dougherty in 1995 and won a five-figure sum in compensation. Frances went into a private hospital in Salisbury to have a large ovarian cyst removed. She found out by chance afterwards from a nurse that a hysterectomy had been performed as well as the removal of both ovaries, fallopian tubes and cervix.

Source: Daily Mail

Albert Singer, Portland Hospital, London

In 1995 widower Michael Silverman won substantial damages for the death in 1992 of his forty-nine year old wife, Ruth, at the private Portland Hospital where she was admitted to have an abdominal hysterectomy. Her bowel was punctured during surgery. Lack of equipment at the hospital meant that she had to be moved to the University College Hospital, but septicaemia had set in and she died. Mr Silverman has since died.

Sources: *Independent, The Lancet, The Times*

Anthony Kenney, Churchill Clinic, London

In 1995 Fouzel Abbas sued gynaecologist Anthony Kenney for negligence for the loss of her reproductive organs at the private Churchill Clinic, found to be due to a mistake caused by the incorrect labelling of tissue samples sent from Pakistan. Mrs Abbas was 21 when she was wrongly diagnosed as having cancer. Her womb, ovaries, cervix and fallopian tubes were removed. She said that she never gave Mr Kenney permission to perform a hysterectomy. Mrs Abbas lost the case.

Source: *Daily Mail*

Leonie Penna, St George's Hospital, Tooting

Shaheen Khan, aged thirty-nine, died at St George's Hospital, Tooting in 1995 after an abdominal hysterectomy in which her artery was punctured. A report into the failure said that 'the management in the post-operative period was below what might reasonably be expected'.

Sources: *Guardian, The Times, Daily Mirror*

Michael Muldoon, Grimsby Hospital Trust

In 1988, Michael Muldoon, Consultant Gynaecologist at Grimsby District General Hospital terminated the pregnancy of Barbara Downer, aged thirty-six, without consent whilst performing a D&C.

THE CASE AGAINST HYSTERECTOMY

Grimsby Hospital Trust

Carol Richardson died as a result of an endometrial re-section in which an artery was pierced. An investigation revealed a 'poor standard of surgical care'. Her family received £5,000 compensation.

Kay Hallberg died as a result of an endometrial ablation in which four perforations were made to the uterus and the bowel which were not competently dealt with. Peritonitis set in leading to progressive failure of the kidneys, liver, heart and lungs. She was removed to intensive care at the St James Hospital in Leeds but she died eighteen days later. The coroner referred to a 'cascade of medical catastrophe' and that 'the standard of medical care fell below the level required'.

Source: BBC Face the Facts

Ian Ferguson, St Thomas's Hospital, London

In 1992 Caroline Richmond, aged fifty-one, went into St Thomas's as a patient of top gynaecologist, Ian Ferguson, to have an endometrial ablation. Ferguson did not perform the operation he had consent for, and instead decided to perform a full hysterectomy and oophorectomy. She reported this to the police who investigated the case, but the Crown Prosecution Service could not establish enough evidence to bring a case against the hospital.

Sources: Independent, Daily Express

Timothy Spencer, Isaac Manyonda, St Peter's Hospital, Chertsey

Sandra Simkin, aged fifty-one, was diagnosed as having an ovarian cyst in 1993 which she wanted to have removed. But Isaac Manyonda, the Gynaecological Registrar, told her that cancer could not be ruled out, so the only operation they would do would be to remove all the organs. She refused, but her GP threatened to 'wash his hands of her' if she did not agree to it. She found out one year after the operation that it had been totally unnecessary.

Sources: Daily Mail, Observer, Woman's Realm

GYNAECOLOGY IN THE NEWS

Campaigning for better treatment: proposal for a Women's Medical Protection Act

When I discovered that the operation I was pressurised into having was so completely unnecessary I was shocked and devastated. I just could not believe that this had happened in the United Kingdom. Ideas about justice were swimming around my head. I felt that I had been robbed of something priceless for no reason at all. When I tried to find out why, I came up against brick walls, doors were metaphorically slammed in my face; I was subject to abrupt telephone conversations and dismissive comments, and treated like a fool.

My first reaction was one of deep despair and I suffered terrible depression. My next feeling was one of rage – how dare they do this to me? And I raged for a long time and met many other women who were angry too. I began to see that this was a much bigger issue – that there were *hundreds* of women in exactly the same situation, women who had been through the same depression and anxiety that I had, women who felt that they had been abused and cast aside as well. My response then changed to one of sustained anger and a determination to put things right for other women. Out of this constructive anger has come this book and the Campaign Against Hysterectomy and Unnecessary Operations on Women.

It seems to me that sustained *patient power* could alter things, and that if enough women are prepared to show that they care about this issue then things will most certainly change. I have spoken to many people in medicine, including gynaecologists, and I have done a lot of research in medical papers, and there is support for the views that we women hold about the hysterectomy business.

All the other improvements which women have achieved in liberating themselves have come about through protest and subsequent legislation. For this reason, I have drafted proposals for a Women's Medical Protection Act to protect women against the abuses of doctors and medical care. This campaign is not just for women who have suffered the experience of unnecessary operations; it is for every woman. If you care about what happens to your daughter, your sister, your aunt or your granddaughter, then join the campaign and help us to achieve these much needed changes.

AIMS OF THE CAMPAIGN AGAINST HYSTERECTOMY AND UNNECESSARY OPERATIONS ON WOMEN

This campaign has been set up to right what is a major wrong in society, namely that 90 per cent of all hysterectomies may be unnecessary. We believe that women all over the nation are being robbed of their wombs and ovaries with little concern for the effect it may have on their later health, emotional welfare, and long-term relationships. The campaign aims also to draw attention to other surgical abuses of women, particularly the high number of enforced Caesarean sections, and unnecessary breast surgery.

THE CAMPAIGN SETS OUT TO ACHIEVE THE FOLLOWING GOALS:

1. To draw attention to the present situation through a press and media campaign.

2. To draw public attention to the campaign through rallies and protest marches.

3. To attract members to the campaign and to establish working campaign cells in all parts of the nation.

4. To draw up a petition and collect one quarter of a million signatures demanding appropriate treatment for women by doctors and gynaecologists.

5. To lobby MPs with the purpose of creating a Women's Medical Protection Act, setting out limitations to the power of surgeons and gynaecologists, making mandatory provisions for second expert opinions to all proposals for surgery, and counselling for all patients and their partners both before and after surgery.

6. To create an effective pressure group which will change the abusive culture surrounding women's healthcare and to provide a choice of access to female medical practitioners in this sector of medicine.

7. To encourage the government to assign certain hospitals, approved by the campaign because of their caring attitude to women, to be specialist hospitals for gynaecological or other surgery.

8. To produce truthful literature about the various operations and their consequences so that women are properly informed.

9. To pressurise the government to authorise the distribution of truthful literature to all adult female patients so that women can make informed decisions about their healthcare.

10. To encourage all General Practitioners to take an active and informed interest in women's healthcare and to play a major role in prescribing treatments.

PROPOSAL FOR A WOMEN'S MEDICAL PROTECTION ACT

The Women's Medical Protection Act aims to redress four surgical abuses of women:

- Unnecessary hysterectomies (removal of the womb and cervix)
- Unecessary oophorectomies (removal of the ovaries)
- Unnecessary Caesarean sections
- Unnecessary breast operations and mastectomies

The Act makes it mandatory that no surgery is to be carried out without the explicit consent of the patient. The surgeon may not use 'clinical judgement' or any other stated reason to remove the reproductive organs and breasts of women without the explicit knowledge and approval of the patient. Should the surgeon in the course of an operation remove these organs without consent for whatever reason, the surgeon will be deemed to have committed an offence in law.

The Act makes it mandatory that a pregnant woman is given every opportunity to have a normal delivery without the interference of gynaecologists and without being forced to have a Caesarean section. Any gynaecologist performing a Caesarean section against the explicit wish of the patient will have committed an offence in law of assault against the patient.

The Act makes it mandatory that the patient and her spouse or partner be counselled by trained counsellors as to the outcome of any operation on a woman's reproductive organs, its psychological and emotional effects and its effect on sexual relations and partnership relations. The counsellor's role is to advise the patient of her rights in law and interpret medical information for her. The counsellor is to be present with the patient at all meeting with the gynaecologist and is required to advise the patient of her rights. The counsellor's role is to ensure that the patient's consent to surgery is truly *informed* consent.

The Act makes it mandatory that the patient have a second specialist opinion for her condition. The patient is to be presented with all reports of tests and examinations so that she is fully informed about her condition. The counsellor is to be present at all times with the surgeon to interpret and explain the reports and documents presented to her.

The Act makes it mandatory that the consent form be signed and witnessed before entering the hospital and in the presence of the counsellor and the surgeon. The patient may revoke the consent form at any time before the operation if she decides not to go ahead. The consent form shall also indicate that the patient has received counselling and that all documents and reports pertinent to her case have been shown to her.

It is mandatory that no Caesarean section, no breast surgery, no mastectomy, no hysterectomy, no oophorectomy or removal of the cervix be performed unless the operation is necessary for medical reasons alone. The conditions determining necessity are as follows:

Caesarean section	Only if the mother wants the operation or there is no other way to ensure the health of the mother and child. The Act requires a second mandatory expert opinion.
Mastectomy/ Breast surgery	That there is the *proved* presence of cancer cells. The Act requires a second expert opinion.
Hysterectomy	That there is the *proved* presence of cancer cells, or that all other treatments have been tried and have failed. The Act requires a second mandatory expert opinion.

THE CASE AGAINST HYSTERECTOMY

Cervix	That there is the *proved* presence of cancer cells. The Act requires a second expert opinion.
Oophorectomy	That there is the *proved* presence of cancer cells. The Act requires a second expert opinion.

The Act makes provision for the treatment of gynaecological problems and breast surgery only in licensed specialist medical centres. One NHS Hospital in London is to be established as an exclusive and specialist centre for women's health, for gynaecological and breast surgery, and to co-ordinate and set uniform standards of practice for the whole of NHS. This centre is also to be the national training centre for gynaecology, obstetrics and breast surgery. A number of designated regional medical centres are also to be licensed as specialist medical centres, operating under the direction and standards laid down by the London Hospital. These hospitals are to be provided with the specialist equipment guaranteed to ensure a high level of patient care. Private hospitals can apply for a licence to practise surgery providing they comply with the conditions set down.

The Act makes mandatory the preservation of women's breasts and sexual organs provided that the presence of cancer does not justify invasive surgery or surgical removal, or there is no alternative treatment. In place of hysterectomy will be myomectomy, endometrial treatments and removal or aspiration of benign cysts. Only the latest surgical techniques devised to preserve the organs are to be used. Those practitioners who remain in gynaecology are to be fully trained in the new techniques.

CAMPAIGN AGAINST HYSTERECTOMY AND UNNECESSARY OPERATIONS ON WOMEN CONSENT FORM

AGREEMENT TO SURGERY BETWEEN PATIENT AND DOCTOR/AND NHS TRUST

I _____ agree to have an

operation for _____

consisting of the following procedure _____

at _____ Hospital on (day) _____ (month) _____ (year) _____

This agreement is made only insofaras the procedure described above, and no other procedure or treatment is agreed to by me. Should the surgeon/gynaecologist decide to perform any other procedure during the course of the operation, this is done expressly *against* my wishes and the outcome of that action will be legal action against the gynaecologist/surgeon and the hospital.

Should the surgeon/gynaecologist discover in the course of performing this procedure that another treatable condition exists then the only action *acceptable to me* is to perform the procedure described above, and to tell me about the outcome and diagnosis *when I am conscious* or to abandon the operation until further surgical options can be discussed with me. I only give consent to additional surgery if such surgery will save my life and without it I would die.

Copies of this agreement to be distributed to the attached list as follows:

_____ Gynaecologist/Surgeon _____ GP

_____ Patient's Solicitor

_____ Chief Executive of the Hospital Trust

_____ Patient giving consent to hospital

Signed _____ Patient _____ Name (capitals)

Signed _____ Witness _____ Name (capitals)

Signed _____ Witness _____ Name (capitals)

(Day) _____ (Month) _____ (Year) _____

Where to go for advice and help: Organisations and helplines

THE ARMARANT TRUST
11–13 Charterhouse Buildings
London EC1M 7AN
Telephone: 0171 608 3222
  Membership: £20 per year (cheque payable to Amarant Services).
  Information Pack £5.
  The Amarant Trust is an independent medical charity aimed at promoting a better understanding of the menopause and hormone replacement therapy. The Trust operates a fully equipped clinic where patients can obtain a completely confidential examination for under £100.
  The Trust operates a 24-hour helpline of recorded advice on the menopause, HRT and Osteoporosis: telephone 0891 660 620 – 39 pence per minute
  For members of the Trust there is a helpline service provided by a trained nurse.

AVMA (ACTION FOR VICTIMS OF MEDICAL NEGLIGENCE)
Bank Chambers
1 London Road
Forest Hill
London SE23 3TP

AVMA was set up by playwright and author Peter Rawnsley as a result of writing a television play, a true story about a woman who suffered a bowel puncture as a result of a laparoscopic sterilisation. The hundreds of letters he received following the screening of the play pointed to a social problem and AVMA was set up as a consequence in 1982. AVMA helps people who have become victims of medical accidents and this includes any action by a doctor which has led to an adverse effect on the patient. AVMA provides help for both legal and non-legal work. It advises patients on how to make a complaint and recommends them to expert medical litigation solicitors. A patient sends details of their complaint to AVMA who assigns it to a caseworker to act on his/her behalf, checking the progress of the solicitor, and providing names of potential expert witnesses.

BRITISH ACUPUNCTURE COUNCIL
Park House
206 Latimer Road
London W10 6RE
Telephone: 0181 964 0222

List of practitioners free.

Acupuncture is an ancient system of medicine which works on the whole body. It corrects hormonal imbalances and is particularly good for helping with the effects and pain of endometriosis and painful periods.

BRITISH ASSOCIATION FOR COUNSELLING
1 Regent Place
Rugby
Warks CV21 2PJ
Telephone: 01788 578 328 (Information)
01788 550 899 (Administration)

List of counsellors available in your local area available on receipt of A4 SAE.

Directory of counsellors for the United Kingdom available for £25.

BRITISH ASSOCIATION FOR SEXUAL AND MARITAL THERAPY
PO Box 62
Sheffield S10 3TS

List of therapists available on application.

The Association was set up to promote research into sexual functioning and therapy. Maintains a register of therapists. Information brochure provided to enquirers. Holds conferences and meetings.

BRITISH HOMEOPATHIC ASSOCIATION
27A Devonshire Street
London W1N 1RJ
Telephone: 0171 935 2163

Free information pack on receipt of SAE.

Maintains a list of homeopathic doctors and hospitals, and produces leaflets on different conditions. Has an extensive library available for use by the public.

BRITISH MEDICAL ASSOCIATION
BMA House
Tavistock Square
London WC1H 9JP
Telephone: 0171 387 4499

Limited information service available on doctors and organisations.

The doctors' professional association promotes medicine and its allied sciences and is a pressure group to promote the improvement of community health. The BMA publishes the *British Medical Journal* and a number of specialist medical publications, as well as papers on current health issues. It is responsible for raising awareness of health risks involved in current practice and in society in general, and for setting guidelines for doctors on medical ethics and consent to surgery.

CAMPAIGN AGAINST HYSTERECTOMY AND UNNECESSARY OPERATIONS ON WOMEN
PO Box 300
Woking, Surrey
GU22 0YE
Telephone: 01483 715435
Helpline: 9.30 a.m. to 12.30 p.m., Wednesday to Sunday.

Membership £10 per year, £7 for pensioners and those on social security payments.

The Campaign was set up to stop the abuse of unnecessary hysterectomies. The campaign is promoting The Women's Medical Protection Act to protect all women from the abuse of unnecessary operations. It provides regular bulletins for members, an annual newspaper and annual conference. It has five regional spokespeople and four 'expert' committees – Medical Information; Law and Consent; Administration and Sponsorship; and a Legal Fund Committee.

COMMUNITY HEALTH COUNCILS
You can find the telephone number of your local CHC by looking under Community Health Council in your local telephone directory.

Community Health Councils were set up under the National Health Service Reorganisation Act 1973 to act as the 'patient's friend' in the case of a complaint against an NHS hospital or doctor. The Community Health Councils are completely independent of the NHS. The Council officers will help you with your complaint against your hospital, doctor, GP and dentist. They will listen to your case, accompany you to any meetings with the Chief Executive of the Hospital or Health Services Authority and/or gynaecologist, and act as your support in these meetings. They will help to get your hospital records and notes and advise on legal redress. They are linked with AVMA.

COUNCIL OF COMPLEMENTARY AND ALTERNATIVE MEDICINE
Park House
206 Latimer Road
London W10 6RE
Telephone: 0171 237 5165
Will send an information pack on therapies on receipt of SAE. (29p stamp) and a cheque for £1.50.

The council, established since1985, in concerned with the promotion, training and safety of four alternative therapies – acupuncture, osteopathy, medical herbalism and homeopathy. It is a pressure group to gain acceptability for these therapies within the NHS and medicine generally, so that they will be offered to patients along with surgical and traditional medical therapies.

THE ENDOMETRIOSIS SOCIETY
50 Westminster Palace Gardens
1–7 Artillery Row
London SW1P 1RL
Telephone: 0171 222 2776
National helpline from 7 p.m. to 10 p.m. every day, including bank holidays.

Membership: £12 per year individual members, £10 associate members, £7 to those on social security benefits.

The society was founded to help sufferers of endometriosis, to raise funds for research and to create awareness of this chronic condition. The society produces a newsletter and number of books and leaflets about endometriosis, surgical and hormone treatments, fertility, and complementary therapies. It has a medical panel to investigate individual members' problems and it runs regular workshops about endometriosis and related subjects.

FAMILY PRACTITIONER SERVICES AUTHORITY
You can obtain the address of your local family Practitioner Services Authority from your public library information service.

Every health region has a family Practitioner Services Authority to whom you can address any complaint against your GP. The authority is obliged to investigate all complaints and report on them. Complaints have to be received within thirteen weeks of the patient first becoming aware of the problem, but the authority can investigate 'out of time' complaints providing the reason for the delay is acceptable to the Authority. If the patient is not happy with the decision of the authority there is an appeals procedure.

GENERAL MEDICAL COUNCIL
44 Hallam Street
London W1N 6AE
Telephone: 0171 580 7642
The General Medical is a council of doctors and lay people set up by law and its powers are defined in the Medical Act 1983. Its duties are designed to protect the interests of patients, including maintaining a register of qualified doctors and dealing with complaints against doctors. The GMC is the body which decides whether a doctor should remain on the medical register, and therefore be able to practise medicine, if convicted of a criminal offence or found guilty of professional misconduct. The GMC can consider a complaint from anyone and there is no time limit within which a complaint must be made. The complaint is considered by two committees, the Preliminary Proceedings Committee and the Professional Conduct Committee. The Preliminary Proceedings Committee, which meets three times a year in private, considers a sworn statement of complaint and the doctor's written comments. If the Preliminary Committee decides not to refer the case to the Professional Conduct Committee it may send a letter of warning or advice to the doctor about his or her professional conduct. The Professional Conduct Committee meets in March, July and November or December of each year to consider complaints; its proceedings are held in public and are similar to those of a criminal court.

HEALTH SERVICES OMBUDSMAN
The Health Service Commissioner for
England
Church House
Great Smith Street
London SW1P 3BW
Telephone: 0171 276 2035 or 0171 276
3000

**THE HEALTH SERVICE COMMISSIONER
FOR SCOTLAND**
Second Floor
11 Melville Crescent
Edinburgh EH3 7LU
Telephone: 0131 225 7465

**THE HEALTH SERVICE COMMISSIONER
FOR WALES**
4th Floor
Pearl Assurance House
Greyfriars Road
Cardiff CF1 3AG
Telephone: 0122 239 4621

The Health Services Ombudsman was
set up to investigate complaints against
the administration of the health service
and its prime role is to see that the
complaints procedure is properly and
effectively administered. It has a
supervisory and 'last port of call' role in
dealing with complaints about hospitals
and doctors; but it has a more direct role,
which it has taken over from the Family
Practitioner Appeals Board, in dealing
with complaints about GPs. The
Ombudsman's role has been recently
strengthened to include clinical
complaints as well as complaints about
maladministration.

**THE INSTITUTE FOR COMPLEMENTARY
MEDICINE**
PO Box 194
London SE16 1QZ
Information on 18 divisions of
Complementary medicine available in
receipt of SAE and 2 19p or 25p stamps.
The institute covers a number of
therapies which are beneficial to women
with gynaecological problems –
aromatherapy, healing/counselling,
nutrition, reflexology, remedial massage
and Chinese medicine. The institute
promotes complementary medicine as a
stand-alone technique or in conjunction
with traditional medicine and co-
ordinates and sets standards of practice.

**THE LAW SOCIETY MEDICAL NEGLIGENCE
PANEL**
Law Society's Halls
113 Chancery Lane
London WC2A 1PL
Telephone: Freephone 0500 192 939
Provides a list of medical negligence
solicitors to enquirers.

LIBERTY
The National Council for Civil Liberties
21 Tabard Street
London SE1 4LA
0171 403 3888
Membership: £20 individual £25
double, students/pensioners £6 single
£10 double, Prisoner £3 per year.
Liberty campaigns for a society built
on democratic participation of all its
members, based on openness, the right
to dissent, and respect for diversity. It
aims to secure the equal rights and
liberties of everyone and oppose any
abuse or excessive use of power. Liberty
is active in eighteen areas where liberty
or rights are being restricted: this
includes women's and health rights.
Liberty actively investigates rights and
abuses in society and produces studies
of its researches. It is a formidable
pressure group for change. It has a
comprehensive publications list, and
organises conferences and festivals.

**THE NATIONAL COUNCIL OF WOMEN OF
GREAT BRITAIN**
36 Danbury Street
London N1
Telephone: 0171 354 2395
Individual membership: £25 per year
payable to NCWGB.
Link membership for organisations
£10.
The NCW aims at improving the
quality of life for all women and is linked
with a number of groups dedicated to
serving women, and is a platform for
change. It has a national network of
branches and regions. It commissions
research into matters of importance to
women. Annual conference.

NATIONAL INSTITUTE OF MEDICINAL HERBALISTS
56 Longbrook Street
Exeter
Devon EX4 6AH
Telephone: 01392 426022
General information about medicinal herbalism and a register of members will be supplied on receipt of SAE. (29p)

THE NATIONAL OSTEOPOROSIS SOCIETY
PO Box 10
Radstock
Bath BA3 3YB
Telephone: 01761 432 472
Helpline: 01761 431 594
Membership: £15 per year, £10 to diagnosed osteoporosis sufferers, £20–£34 per year to healthcare workers.

NOS is an independent registered charity aimed at raising awareness of osteoporosis, carrying out research into the condition and ensuring that there is adequate funding for its detection and treatment. The society produces a number of pamphlets and books on osteoporosis. It provides a telephone helpline staffed by specialist nurses, individual replies from medical experts to individual enquiries, local support groups, newsletters, two free booklets and access to leading specialists at the society's annual conference.

THE PATIENTS SOCIETY
8 Guildford Street
London WC1N 1DT
Telephone: 0171 242 3460
Membership: £12 per year single, £14 per year double membership.

Founded in 1963, the society is a voice for patients which is independent of government, health professionals and the drugs industry. Its aim is to develop the interests, rights and well-being of users and potential users of the health services of the United Kingdom. It has been a powerful pressure group for bringing improvements and change to the NHS. The society provides advice to individuals about non-medical problems, and produces leaflets and brochures of interest to patients. It also produces a quarterly newsletter.

PHARMACEUTICAL SOCIETY OF GREAT BRITAIN
1 Lambeth High Street
London SE1 7JN
Telephone: 0171 735 9141
Provides general information but advises patients to go to their pharmacist for detailed information about the drugs prescribed by their doctors.

The Pharmaceutical Society is the professional body for practising pharmacists.

RIGHTS OF WOMEN
52-54 Featherstone Street
London EC1Y 8RT
Telephone: 0171 251 6577
Free publications list to enquirers.

Rights of Women is an umbrella organisation for several women's organisations concerned with women's rights. It is primarily concerned with helping women to achieve justice in areas such as rape and domestic violence. ROW will help women enquirers to assess whether they have a legal case and find a suitable woman solicitor to handle their case.

THE ROYAL COLLEGE OF SURGEONS OF ENGLAND
35–43 Lincoln's Inn Fields
London WC2A 3PN
Telephone: 0171 405 3474
The Royal College sets standards in surgery and trains doctors, sets examinations and awards diplomas, and provides monitoring and continuing education for doctors. The college has a responsibility to patients and is producing a booklet on consent for patients.

THE SOCIETY FOR MINIMALLY INVASIVE THERAPY
2nd Floor
New Guy's House
Guy's Hospital
St Thomas Street
London SE1
Telephone: 0171 955 5000
Free list of minimally invasive therapists available to enquirers.

The society is dedicated to increasing the amount of minimally invasive surgery performed on patients and will give patients the name of a practitioner of minimally invasive surgery in their area. They have contacts throughout the country. They cite improved recovery time and the reduction of trauma to patients as the reason for recommending minimal surgery.

SUSSEX WOMEN'S SELF-HELP GROUP
32 The Saffrons
Burgess Hill
West Sussex
RH15 8TB
Self-help group of hysterectomy patients who experienced adverse effects from their operations.

WOMEN'S ENDOSCOPIC LASER FOUNDATION
South Cleveland Hospital
Middlesbrough
Cleveland
01642 854 861
Free information pack available to enquirers. Send large SAE, 36p.
South Cleveland Hospital is one of several centres specialising in endoscopic laser treatment and minimal access surgery: the others are The Royal College of Surgeons linked to the Royal Surrey Hospital, Guildford; The Ninewells Hospital, Dundee; and St James's Hospital, Leeds linked to the Leeds Royal Infirmary. The South Cleveland Hospital has pioneered new endometrial treatments in the United Kingdom, especially a new laparoscopic treatment for endometriosis using laser fibres to remove endometrial growths outside the womb. The centre also performs laparoscopic myolysis and myomectomy operations to remove fibroid growths.

WOMEN'S HEALTH
52-54 Featherstone Street
London EC1
Telephone: 0171 251 6580
Helpline: 10 a.m. – 4 p.m. Monday, Wednesday, Thursday and Friday
Free publications list on receipt of SAE (25p).
Women's Health is an organisation dedicated to providing women with truthful information about all of their health problems and recommends both surgical and complementary medicine

where appropriate. Women's Health works with a number of women's groups, including Rights of Women and WNCCC. It has an extensive library on women's health and maintains a database of women's campaigns and help organisations, as well as a listing of women who have had hysterectomies.

WOMEN'S NATIONAL CANCER CONTROL CAMPAIGN
Suna House
128–130 Curtain Road
London EC2A 3AR
Telephone: 0171 729 4688
Helpline: 0171 729 2229 9.30 a.m.– 4.30 p.m.
Free publications on screening for patients, specialist videos available on hire from the campaign.
The WNCCC is a pressure group to support the early diagnosis of breast, cervical and ovarian cancer. The campaign gives advice and support to women who are diagnosed as having cancer. It runs mobile screening units for cervical and breast cancer screening, and provides health days for homeless women. It promotes health and awareness through its talks' programme and publications.

WOMEN'S NUTRITIONAL ADVICE SERVICE
PO Box 268
Lewes
East Sussex BN7 2QN
Telephone: 01273 487366
Cost £30–£98, depending on type of service.
A charity providing information and services to women as part of a complete complementary medicine package. Write in or telephone for information about services. Provides a tailor-made programme of diet, exercise and supplements based on the analysis of a detailed personal questionnaire and a thirty-minute telephone consultation. Patients can have a sixty-minute consultation at their London, Lewes or Hove clinics or a six-month course. Other services included are publications on all aspects of nutrition and women's health and exercise videos. WNAS is actively encouraging women to seek a nutritional solution to menopausal symptoms instead of HRT

Notes

CHAPTER I: STATISTICAL JUSTIFICATION AND CONTRADICTIONS

1   Estimated figure: approximately 74,000 are perfomed in the National Health
     Service each year. For every three performed in the NHS, one is done privately
     (Kings Fund estimate): Hospital Episode Statistics V. 1. Consultant episodes by
     diagnosis, operation and speciality, 1995.

2   Office of Population Censuses and Surveys (OPCS): Registrations of newly
     diagnosed cases of cancer 1990 (provisional) sex, major site and age: England
     and Wales: NHS in Scotland 1993/4: Northern Ireland Cancer Registry
     (estimate).

3   OPCS: Underlying Cause of Death 1993, England and Wales, Table 3 Series DH2
     no 20: Registrar General for Scotland Annual Report 1994: Northern Ireland
     Causes of Death 1994.

4   Vikki Hufnagel, *No More Hysterectomies*, Thorsons, 1988, p. 111.

5   Imperial Cancer Research Fund; Five Year Survival – England and Wales.
     Patients diagnosed in 1981, 10 most survivable cancers.

6   Office of Population Censuses and Surveys (OPCS): Registrations of newly
     diagnosed cases of cancer 1990 (provisional) sex, major site and age, England
     and Wales: NHS in Scotland 1993/4: Northern Ireland Cancer Registry
     (estimate).

7   Imperial Cancer Research Fund: Ovarian Cancer Treatment, Fact Sheet, July
     1995.

8   ibid.

9   OPCS: Underlying Cause of Death 1993, England and Wales, Table 3 Series DH2
     no 20. Calculated from statistics on female population 29, 123 million: Registrar
     General for Scotland. Annual Report 1994: Northern Ireland Cancer Registry
     (estimate).

10   ibid.

11   Imperial Cancer Research Fund: op. cit.

12   OPCS: Registration of newly diagnosed cases of cancer 1990 (provisional) sex,
     major site and age, England and Wales: NHS in Scotland 1993/4: Norhtern
     Ireland Cancer Registry (estimate).

13   Imperial Cancer Research Fund: Five Year Survival – England and Wales.
       Patients diagnosed in 1981, 10 most survivable cancers.
14   OPCS: Registrations of newly diagnosed cases of cancer 1990 (provisional) sex,
       major site and age, England and Wales: NHS in Scotland 1993/4: Northern
       Ireland Cancer Registry (estimate).
15   ibid. Figure calculated from OPCS statistics.
16   OPCS: Underlying Cause of Death 1993, England and Wales, Table 3 Series DH2
       no 20: Registrar General for Scotland Annual Report 1994: Northern Ireland
       Causes of Death 1994.
17   ibid.
18   ibid.
19   ibid.
20   Vikki Hufnagel, No More Hysterectomies, Thorsons, 1988, pp. 136–153.
21   ibid.
22   Angela Coulter, Klim McPherson and Martin Vessey, Social Science Medicine, 'Do
       British Women undergo too many or too few hysterectomies? V. 27 9, pp.
       987–994.
23   Estimated figure, see note 1.
24   University of Dundee, Centre of Medical Education unpublished study of
       patients at the Ninewells Hospital, Dundee; and Debbie Romney-Alexander,
       Women Only: how to find the help you need, Perspective Health Publications, 1994,
       p. 133.
25   The Lancet V. 341 15 May 1993, letter M. F. Oliver, Wynn Institute and Ian Jacobs
       and David Oram, British Journal of Obstetrics and Gynaecology, Prevention of
       ovarian cancer: a survey of the practice of prophylactic oophorectomy by
       fellows and members of the Royal College of Obstetricians and Gynaecologists,
       1989 V. 96 pp. 510–515.
26   The Lancet 25 August 1973, D. H. Richards Depression after hysterectomy
27   Drug and Therapeutic Bulletin V. 32 No 9 15 September 1994 p. 71 Menorrhagia:
       and British Medical Journal V. 300 16 June 1990 pp. 1,537–1,538 Mangement of
       Menorrhagia: Hysteroscopic techniques offer revolution in treatment.
28   Mims Magazine: The Journal of Prescribing and Therapeutics 15 May 1992,
       Menorrhagia: New Ways to Spare the Scalpel; (Comparison of overall morbidity
       1:1,163 to risk of 1:2,500 without surgery).
29   Northern Ireland Cancer Registry: Cancer death patterns and trends p. 41
       Cancer of the ovary, European countries.
30   University of Dundee, op. cit.
31   Debbie Romney–Alexander. op. cit., Section 1; and Nina Ahmad, Women's
       Realm, 'Hands Off Our Bodies, 7 February 1995.
32   British Medical Journal, V. 308 1 January 1994, Female Castration Controversy
       Deserves Some Attention, Letter from Aileen Clarke, Pam Rowe and Nick Black,
       Department of Public Health and Policy, Health Services Research Unit, London
       School of Hygiene and Tropical Medicine, London University.
33   HMSO, Social Trends, 1994 and data supplied by the AA 1994.
34   ibid.
35   OPCS: Underlying Cause of Death 1993, England and Wales, Table 3 Series DH2
       no: 20: Registrar General for Scotland Annual Report 1994: Northern Ireland
       Causes of Death 1994.
36   ibid.
37   ibid.
38   ibid.
39   HMSO, Social Trends, 1994.
40   ibid.
41   ibid and AA Information, 1994.

42   Angela Coulter, Kim McPherson and Martin Vessey, *Social Science Medicine*, 'Do British Women undergo too many or too few hysterectomies?' V. 27 9 pp. 987–994; and Meridian TV. Serve You Right 10 October 1995.

43   Channel 4 'Dispatches' 31 January 1996

44   OPCS, Underlying Cause of Death 1993, England and Wales, Table 3 Series DH2 no 20: Registrar General for Scotland Annual Report 1994: Northern Ireland Causes of Death 1994.

45   Based on costs of operating on, nursing care and post-operative care of NHS patients and the cost of paying sickness benefit for 60 per cent of all 100,000 patients and for prescriptions of all patients. 90 per cent of 73,517 operations is 66,165 unnecessary NHS operations.

1   Cost of operations for gynaecologist, anaesthetist, operating theatre staff plus use of theatre equipment and provision of specialist equipment = £1,600 per operation. Total = £105.86 million.

2   Cost of 7-day stay in hospital, nursing care, medication in hospital, transfusion service, monitoring equipment, catering, specialist post-operative care and emergency services for cases where things go wrong = £1,200 per patient. Total = £79.4 million.

3   The cost of prescriptions and HRT £8 per prescription x 4 times per year for 10 years for 100,00 patients = £32 million.

4   The cost of employing 70 per cent of gynaecologists unnecesassarily at a salary of £70,000 per year = £49 million.

5   The cost of employing 70 per cent of 1,400 qualified nurses unnecessarily at a salary of £20,000 per year = £19.6 million.

6   The cost of employing 70 per cent of ancillary workers out of 2,100 – porters, cleaners, caterers, receptionists, clerks etc. at a cost of £10,00 per year = £14.7 million.

7   Estimated cost of providing buildings, equipment servicing, overheads, monitoring equipment and buildings, provision of other staff and the training of doctors and nurses = £50 million per year.

8   The cost of providing sickness benefit for an estimated 60 per cent of 100,000 women who work at £47.20 per week for 12 weeks = £34 million.

Total cost to the NHS = £384.56 million per year

CHAPTER 2: ALTERNATIVE SURGICAL TECHNIQUES
AND MEDICAL THERAPIES

1   *Vogue*, November 1994 Take it or leave it? Whose body is it anyway? Claire Merton pp. 37–39.

2   Ian Jacobs and David Oram, *British Journal of Obstetrics and Gynaecology*, Prevention of ovarian cancer: a survey of the practice of prophylactic oophorectomy by fellows and members of the Royal College of Obstetricians and Gynaecologists, 1989 V. 96 pp. 510–515; John Studd and Joan Pitkin, British Menopause Society Conference 1994, 'This house believes that the benefits of castration at hysterectomy outweigh the disadvantages.'

3   Meridian TV, 'Serve You Right', 10 October 1995; and Channel 4 'Dispatches', 31 January 1996.

4   Johannes Vingerling, Ida Dielemans, Jacqueline Witteman, Albert Hoffman, Diederick Grobbee, Paulus de Jong, *British Medical Journal*, Macular degeneration and early menopause: a case-control study, 1995, V. 310 pp. 1570–1571.

5   Channel 4, 'Dispatches', 31 January 1996.

6   This figure is an estimate of all risks, DTB, *Drug and Therapeutics Bulletin* V. 32 no. 9, 15 September 1994 gives a figure for mortality after hysterectomy as 6 per 10,000 which is 1:1,600 for death only. This means that 62 women will die from having a hysterectomy each year.

7   Angela Coulter, Klim McPherson and Martin Vessey, *Social Science Medicine*, 'Do British Women undergo too many or too few hysterectomies?' V. 27 9 pp. 987–994.

8   *British Medical Journal*, V. 308 1 January 1994, Female Castration Controversy Deserves Some Attention, Letter from Aileen Clarke, Pam Rowe and Nick Black, Department of Public Health and Policy, Health Services Research Unit, London School of Hygiene and Tropical Medicine, London University.

9   Angela Coulter et al; op. cit.

10 Felicity Smart and Stuart Campbell, *Fibroids: the latest treatment options for this common problem*, Thorsons, 1993, p. 46.

11 Tony Seeley, *British Medical Journal*, V. 305 3 October 1992, Oestrogen replacement therapy after hysterectomy and Vikki Hufnagel, *No More Hysterectomies*, Thorsons, 1988, p. 48.

12 ibid. pp. 157–63.

CHAPTER 3: THE PHYSIOLOGICAL, PSYCHOLOGICAL AND EMOTIONAL EFFECTS OF HYSTERECTOMY.

1   Vikki Hufnagel, *No More Hysterectomies*, Thorsons, 1988, p. 48.

2   David Alexander et al, *British Medical Journal*, V. 312 3 February 1996 pp. 280–284, Randomised trial comparing hysterectomy with endometrial ablation for dysfunctional uterine bleeding: psychiatric and psychosocial aspects.

3   Channel 4, 'Dispatches', 31 January 1996.

4   Vikki Hufnagel, op. cit., p. 3; *Daily Telegraph*, 23 April 1994; Sybil Shainwald, The Network News, May–June 1985, RX For Your Legal Health: A legal response to hysterectomy abuse.

5   Harold Persky, Lorraine Dreisbach, William Miller, Charles O'Brien, Miftah Khan, Harold Lief, Natalie Charney and Dorothy Strauss, *Psychosomatic Medicine*, September 1982, V. 44 no.4, The Relation of Plasma Androgen Levels to Sexual Behaviours and Attitudes of Women.

6   Lorraine Dennerstein, Carl Wood and Graham Burrows, *Obstetrics and Gynaecology*, 1977, V. 49 1, pp. 92–96 Sexual Response following Hysterectomy and Oophorectomy; D.H. Richards, *The Lancet*, 1973, 25 August 1973, pp. 430–432. Depression after Hysterectomy.

CHAPTER 4: THE EFFECT OF HYSTERECTOMY ON SEX AND RELATIONSHIPS

1   Leon Zussman et al, *American Journal of Obstetrics and Gynaecology*, V. 140 no.7, 1981, Sexual response after hysterectomy-oophorectomy: Recent studies and reconsideration of psychogenesis.

2   Don Sloan, *American Journal of Obstetrics and Gynaecology*, 1978, 131, pp. 598–605, The emotional and psychosexual aspects of hysterectomy.

3   Miriam Stoppard, (ed.) *Woman's Body*, Dorling Kindersley, 1994, p. 129.

4   Vikki Hufnagel, *No More Hysterectomies*, Thorsons, 1988.

CHAPTER 5: AGEING, THE MENOPAUSE, HRT AND HYSTERECTOMY

1   Germaine Greer, *The Change*, Penguin, 1992.

2   HMSO, *Social Trends*, 1994; and *Daily Telegraph*, 9 August 1985.

3   Dr Ellen Grant, *Sexual chemistry: understanding our hormones, the Pill and HRT*, Cedar, 1994.

4   *Chic Magazine*, 1995, 'HRT: who needs it?'

5   Angela Coulter, Kings Fund; and *Daily Telegraph*, 10 November 1994.

CHAPTER 7: GPS AND GYNAECOLOGISTS: THE NATIONAL HEALTH SERVICE AND PRIVATE MEDICINE

1 Kings Fund, 1995.
2 *Guardian*, 24 September 1994, 'Ousted NHS chief attacks poor care'.
3 *Daily Telegraph*, 14 November 1994, 'NHS Trust Manager attacked for saying patients come third'.
4 Radio 4, 1995.
5 *Consumer Reports*, September 1990, V. 55 pp. 603–608, 'Hysterectomy and its alternatives'.

CHAPTER 8: SEEKING REDRESS: THE NHS COMPLAINTS SYSTEM AND CIVIL ACTION IN THE COURTS

1 *The Lancet*, Brewin, Thurstan and the *Daily Telegraph*, 16 June 1994.

CHAPTER 10: WHAT YOU CAN DO TO HELP YOURSELF

1 Dairy Diary analysis of milk value.
2 Alan and Maryon Stewart, Women's Nutritional Advisory Service. Self-help guide; Liz Earle, *Eat Yourself Beautiful*, BBC Books, 1992.
3 Felicity, Smart and Stuart Campbell, *Fibroids: the latest treatment options for this common problem*, Thorsons, 1993.
4 Ellen Grant, *Sexual Chemistry: understanding our hormones, the Pill and HRT*, Cedar, 1994, p. 12.
5 Vikki Hufnagel, *No More Hysterectomies*, Thorsons, 1988, pp. 87–98.
6 ibid., p. 187.
7 This is advocated by some exercise specialists and gynaecological nurses although not proven as a technique to prevent all prolapse conditions.
8 Alan and Maryon Stewart, op. cit.
9 Rina Nissim, *Natural Healing in Gynaecology*, Pandora, 1996.
10 Vikky Hufnagel, op. cit., pp. 94–5.
11 Rina Nissim, op. cit.
12 Ellen Grant, *Sexual Chemistry: understanding our hormones, the Pill and HRT*, Cedar, 1994.
13 Alan and Maryon Stewart, op. cit.
14 ibid.

CHAPTER 11: HYSTERECTOMY ABROAD AND WOMEN'S RIGHTS

1 Lynn Payer, *Medicine and Culture*, Victor Gollancz, 1989, pp. 15–34.
2 ibid., pp. 124–152.
3 Vikki Hufnagel, *No More Hysterectomies*, Thorsons, 1988, p. 60.
4 Angela Coulter, Klim McPherson and Martin Vessey. *Social Science Medicine*, 'Do British Women undergo too many or too few hysterectomies?' V. 27 9, pp. 987–994.
5 ibid., Channel 4, Dispatches, February 1996.
6 Angela Coulter, op. cit.
7 Lynn Payer, *Medicine and Culture*, Victor Gollancz, 1989, pp. 35–73.
8 ibid.
9 Helen Roberts. *Women's Health Counts*, Routledge, 1990, p. 128.
10 Lynn Payer, op. cit., p. 112.
11 ibid., pp. 102–103.
12 ibid., pp. 122–123.
13 ibid.
14 ibid., p. 148.
15 April Carter, *The Politics of Women's Rights*, Longman, 1988, pp.4–5.
16 ibid., p. 6.
17 ibid., pp. 6–7.

NOTES

Recommended reading list

Jan Clark, Hysterectomy and the Alternatives Virago, 1993

Gorman, Teresa and Whitehead, Malcolm The Amarant Book of HRT Pan Books, 1989

Grant, Dr Ellen Sexual Chemistry: Understanding our Hormones, The Pill and HRT Cedar: Reed Books, 1994

Greer, Germaine The Change Penguin, 1992

Hawkridge, Caroline Living with Endometriosis: A Practical Guide to the Causes and Treatments Vermilion, 1996

Hufnagel, Vikki No More Hysterectomies Thorsons, 1988

Llewellyn-Jones, Derek Everywoman: Gynaecology Guide for Life Penguin, 1993

Melville, Arabella Natural Hormone Health Thorsons, 1990

Moran, Diana and Franks, Helen Bone Boosters: Natural Ways to Prevent Osteoporosis Boxtree, 1995

Nissim, Rina Natural Healing in Gynaecology HarperCollins, 1996

Romney-Alexander, Debbie Women Only: How to Find the Help You Need Perspective Health Publications, 1994

Smart, Felicity and Campbell, Stuart Fibroids: The Latest Treatment Options for this Common Problem Thorsons, 1993

Stewart, Maryon Beat the Menopause without HRT Headline, 1995

Wescott, Patsy Alternative Healthcare for Women Thorsons, 1991

Wescott, Patsy Hormone Relacement Therapy: Making Your Own Decision Thorsons, 1993

What Doctors Don't Tell You Monthly newsletter, £29.95 per year. 4 Wallace Road London N1 2PG